Phonological Intervention

Concepts and Procedures

Edited by:

Michael A. Crary

Southern Illinois University—Carbondale, Carbondale

Contributors:

David Ingram

University of British Columbia, Vancouver

Joann Fokes

Ohio University, Athens

Lawrence D. Shriberg

University of Wisconsin—Madison, Madison

Stephen E. Blache

Southern Illinois University—Carbondale, Carbondale

Barbara W. Hodson

San Diego State University, San Diego

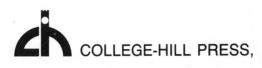

COLLEGE-HILL PRESS,

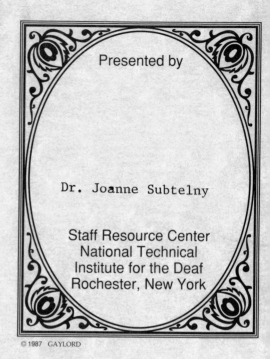

Presented by

Dr. Joanne Subtelny

Staff Resource Center
National Technical
Institute for the Deaf
Rochester, New York

© 1987 GAYLORD

College-Hill Press, Inc.
4284 41st Street
San Diego, California 92105

Library of Congress Cataloging in Publication Data

Phonological intervention, concepts and procedures.

Includes bibliographies and index.
1. Articulation disorders in children—
Congresses. I. Crary, Michael A., 1952–
RJ496.S7P47   618.92'85506   81-21706
ISBN 0-933014-73-2   AACR2

Printed in the United States of America.

1251296

Contents

Contributing Authors

David Ingram, Ph.D.
Department of Linguistics
University of British Columbia
Vancouver, B.C.

Joann Fokes, Ph.D.
School of Hearing and Speech Sciences
Ohio University
Athens, OH

Lawrence D. Shriberg, Ph.D.
Department of Communicative Disorders
University of Wisconsin—Madison
Madison, WI

Stephen E. Blache, Ph.D.
Department of Communication Disorders & Sciences
Southern Illinois University—Carbondale
Carbondale, IL

Barbara W. Hodson, Ph.D.
Department of Communicative Disorders
San Diego State University
San Diego, CA

Preface

During the past decade, speech-language therapists have witnessed trans-formations in the manner in which "articulation disorders" are remediated. In fact, as the reader will experience in the following pages, the term "artic-ulation disorders" has been challenged and, for many of us, has been replaced by the term "phonological disorders." This change of focus has resulted not only from influences from linguistic science, but also, from a change in the type of clients receiving speech-language services. From cer-tain perspectives, this transformation has been rapid. Many clinicians have been confused by a plethora of articles, monographs, and tests—each advocating an apparently different approach to intervention with unintelli-gible children! Questions such as "What should I be evaluating?" and "What should I work on?" have not been uncommon in reference to children with "multiple articulation errors." These are valid clinical questions. They deserve practical and plausible responses. The pages which follow directly address these issues in a format beneficial to practicing speech-language clinicians and to students who will someday be facing similar problems.

Phonological Intervention: Concepts and Procedures is the outgrowth of an exceptional meeting that was held in May, 1980. That meeting, entitled "The First Major Conference on Phonological Disorders in Children," brought together a group of people who have been leaders in the area of phono-logical disorders. The intent of that meeting was to address the issues just mentioned. The result was a two-and-a-half day conference in which speakers and participants shared both concepts and procedures relevant to clinical intervention with children presenting phonological disorders. Following the meeting, I received multiple requests for transcripts from those who had attended and, also, from individuals who had heard reports of what had tran-spired. Given the amount of time that has passed since that meeting, it would be unfair to readers to publish a strict transcription. Recognizing this fact, the contributors agreed to follow their respective presentation formats, but to include new developments that have originated since that time. In one respect, this delay has resulted in a more comprehensive book. As readers will soon recognize, the authors of the enclosed chapters have not been idle in the past year. Three have published major books or clinical tools, and all have published articles relevant to phonological disorders in children.

For me, the publication of the manuscript reflects the completion of a special project started two years ago. I would like to thank David Ingram, Joann Fokes, Larry Shriberg, Steve Blache, and Barbara Hodson for their support and contributions. They are truly outstanding, not only as scholars or clinicians, but as individuals. Too, I would like to thank College-Hill Press for providing the avenue by which I was able to finalize this project. Finally, I would like to thank my family, Coleen, Shawn, and "unborn," who tolerated me during these final days of manuscript preparation.

mac

Introduction

In working with children demonstrating multiple articulation errors, clinicians must develop intervention strategies different from traditional sound-by-sound approaches. I have worked with many clinicians who professed frustration over the lack of progress demonstrated by "unintelligible" children. Common problems include not knowing "where to start," "which technique to use," or the lack of carry over—"He can say the sound but doesn't use it in words!" In addressing these issues I have often encouraged clinicians to change their entire approach to intervention in such cases by focusing more on how sound systems are organized than on how individual sounds are produced (or misproduced). Clinicians who follow this advice will find many recent, but scattered, publications promoting a particular assessment or remediation technique along the lines of phonological intervention. After developing a few basic phonological concepts and attempting one or more of these procedures, clinicians often report greater success in these severe cases. The chapters which follow represent a collection of concepts and procedures followed by five experienced professionals in the area of phonological disorders.

Perhaps the best way to introduce this book is to re-introduce the chapter contributors. I say "re-introduce" because each is already well-known for contributions to speech-language pathology.

David Ingram may be best known to clinicians as a result of his 1976 book, *Phonological Disability in Children*. Perhaps more than any other, this book incorporates the term "phonological processes" into our vocabulary. Dr. Ingram's work has had great influence on the clinical management of phonological disorders. At the 1980 conference, Dr. Ingram outlined several questions relevant to the analysis of child speech and, in 1981, he published his procedural guide for speech analysis. In the first chapter of the present text, Dr. Ingram re-addresses questions regarding speech analysis and summarizes his approach.

In Chapter Two, Joann Fokes reviews several issues relevant to the analysis of child speech. Dr. Fokes authored the "Fokes Sentence Builder" and is well-known to clinicians. Too, she has been an early leader in the development of the phonemic contrast approach to therapy for phonologically disordered children. Her chapter presents a detailed review of potential sources of variability in child speech. In this chapter, Dr. Fokes addresses both theorists and practitioners. She demonstrates that both points of view face similar limitations and that each has information valuable to the other. This chapter ends with a presentation of procedures used in phonemic contrast therapy and a discussion of how this approach is appropriate for reducing or eliminating many sources of variability in child speech. Her frequent use of specific examples from clinical experiences provides a functional reality to this chapter.

In Chapter Three, Lawrence Shriberg presents a comprehensive approach to the assessment of phonologically disordered children. This chapter begins by introducing the focal shift from articulatory to phonological disorders. Along these lines, Dr. Shriberg presents background referencing his approach to natural process analysis. He then proceeds through a step-by-step development of his comprehensive diagnostic approach. This is an excellent chapter for clinicians in that it places phonological disorders in perspective with reference to the complete diagnostic battery. Dr. Shriberg's activity in professional journals is well-known. In addition, he has published (*Natural Process Analysis*, 1980) and is developing future texts in the area of phonetics and phonological disorders. His approach to phonological disorders will continue to have a major impact on our profession.

Chapter Four, by Stephen Blache, depicts a slightly different focus in the management of phonological disorders. Dr. Blache's presentation and expansion of the Jakobsonian concept of distinctive features is known to clinicians and theorists through his 1978 text, *The Acquisition of Distinctive Features*. In this present chapter, he reviews the "semantic and pragmatic aspects of the phoneme." Through a series of simple practice exercises, Dr. Blache introduces clinicians to a practical approach to distinctive feature analysis and intervention. He addresses issues varying from identifying target errors to using the distinctive feature approach in establishing homogeneous groups for intervention. Furthermore, this chapter discusses the normal sequence of distinctive feature acquisition upon which his approach is based. Finally, Dr. Blache presents a detailed discussion of "minimal word pairs" as a therapeutic technique.

Barbara Hodson contributes the last chapter of this text. Dr. Hodson has developed a very interesting approach to the remediation of severe phonological disorders in which a child is exposed to several cycles reflecting different goals of phonological organization. Dr. Hodson begins her chapter by describing her view of "low levels of phonological performance." As a result of this introduction, the reader is given a description of her recently published test, "The Assessment of Phonological Processes." Following the description of diagnostic issues, this chapter discusses the identification of remediation priorities and concludes with a detailed presentation of her therapy approach and specific techniques. Those who have enjoyed Dr. Hodson's workshops in the area of phonological disorders will find this chapter an "evolved update" of her continuing work. First-time readers will benefit greatly from the clinical experience behind the development of this approach.

All of these chapters are written in an informal, personalized style that reflects their origin in the 1980 conference. The information in each chapter is up-to-date, and often looks to the future. Readers will notice that the progression of chapters follows a mild trend from concepts to procedures. That is to say that the emphasis on procedures grows slightly in the later chapters. Further, this framework is also followed in each individual chapter. The intent of the book is the lucid presentation of major approaches to the management of phonological disorders. Each chapter, and the book as a whole, reflects the synthesis of concepts and procedures. The title is a simple outgrowth of this synthesis: *Phonological Intervention: Concepts and Procedures.*

1 The Assessment of Phonological Disorders in Children: The State of the Art

David Ingram

Despite all of our scientific efforts, phonological analysis and intervention with disordered children remains very much an 'art.' It is an area that requires creative skill in determining a child's phonological system and insight into how to initiate improvement. In this paper, I will attempt to specify some of the gains we have made in recent years in making such judgements more explicit, and outline some of the decisions we face in the construction of efficient analytic procedures. The discussion should help introduce the diverse approaches presented in this volume, and provide a basis for comparison and evaluation.

The last decade has been one of active research in the area of phonological disorders. I offer the following summary of the status of this area of study:

1. The interest of research has shifted from *articulation* to *phonology*.
2. The data base on normal acquisition and its variation has increased to the point that we have a good descriptive idea of what children do.
3. Comparisons of disordered children to normal ones indicate that both groups follow similar developmental paths.
4. Efforts are concentrating on developing analytic procedures for assessment and intervention with phonologically disordered children.

The shift from articulation to phonology is one of placing articulation in the context of the linguistic system. For example, to say that a child cannot produce "f" depends crucially on whether one is referring strictly to articulation in general, or articulation within a linguistic system. The phonologist is not just concerned with whether or not "f" is produced, but also with target sounds and the contrastive status of substitutions. A child may produce [p] for /f/ (adult "f"), yet produce [f] for /θ/. Also, the [p] for /f/ will result in the loss of certain contrasts which need to be considered when intervention is planned. Articulation is still important, of course, but as part of the functioning of the child's linguistic system.

The descriptive base of data on child phonology has also grown in recent years (c.f. Yeni-Komshian, Kavanaugh, and Ferguson, 1976). This is not to say, of course, that a comprehensive theory exists, but that we do have an idea of the order of appearance of specific patterns of development (see reviews in Shriberg and Kwiatkowski, 1980; and Ingram, 1976). It is this state of affairs, in fact, that has led researchers to attempt more explicit analytic procedures. Also, comparisons between normal and disordered children indicate that disordered children look like younger normal ones, so that the use of normal data for analytic purposes is appropriate. Such research indicates further that the really interesting issue is how all children differ from each other, not how normal and disordered children compare.

The focus of this chapter is on the development of analytic procedures such as those discussed in the present volume. Such approaches allow for consistent assessments of individual children, a crucial step in the development of valid clinical tools for remediation. We need, therefore, to be able to evaluate alternative approaches critically, and understand exactly how they differ from one another. In the next section, I will outline three decisions that underlie the development of any analytic procedure. After, I will present data that exemplify how different decisions can result in different analyses of a child's phonological system. Finally, I will offer some suggestions on how I have made these decisions in my own work (Ingram, 1981).

Three Decisions in Phonological Analysis

The first step involved in any analysis is to answer the following question: *Decision 1:* "What is the *goal* of the analysis?" This has to do with the selection of the units to be studied. In phonological analysis, we can choose among any of the following: individual speech sounds, distinctive features, substitutions, and phonological processes. There are assessment procedures that look at each of these as well as selected combinations.

In making this decision, there are certain assumptions that follow. One of these concerns how *comprehensive* one wishes to be. We all know, for example, that clinicians often work under severe time limitations, and often do not have time to assess all aspects of a child's system. Sometimes, therefore, specific goals are selected because they are felt to be more important than others in determining what is most in need of change. While this is a significant pragmatic factor, it is also important to consider that a truly comprehensive and satisfactory analysis may not be reducible to a predetermined period of one or two hours. We always need to consider what a particular goal actually tells us about the child's entire system.

A second assumption behind this decision is that the goal of the analysis is *psychologically real*. For example, the selection of distinctive features or phonological processes assumes that these are units which speakers use in the organization of language. The psychological reality of these units, as well as others, however, is not necessarily established. The evidence by-and-large consists of theoretical analysis of how languages seem to work.

Even if the units selected are psychologically real, there is the further assumption that their specification in turn will *predict change*. The value in finding a particular unit is in being able to initiate change in the child's system by working on that unit. For example, a phonological process such as stopping of fricatives can be predictive if one claims that the appearance of one fricative will lead to others. If fricative acquisition is gradual, however, as appears to be the case (c.f. Ingram et al., 1981), then the predictive value is limited. One can claim that the processes isolate what should be easier for the child, with no predictions of generalization. This latter position appears to underlie current clinical suggestions based on phonological processes. (See Ingram, 1976, Chapter 6 for a similar discussion regarding distinctive features.)

After the selection of a goal, we next have to decide what will be the data for analysis. This leads us to our second major decision. *Decision 2:* "What is appropriate data for analysis?" Here, the choices include the use of a spontaneous sample, word elicitation, and imitation. Each has its advantages and disadvantages. As pointed out by Shriberg and Kwiatkowski (1980), standard articulation tests use words that are complex and difficult for young children and thereby undermine the child's actual ability. These authors thus recommend the use of spontaneous samples. Such samples, however, usually do not yield a wide range of vocabulary so that some word prompting is also included.

Regardless of the sampling procedure, there are further decisions about what data to include in an analysis. One is whether one production of a word is sufficient. Since children's productions are variable, it may be that one production may not be the one that the child typically uses. This point relates to another concerning the number of words that should be used to test a specific sound. Some tests use just one word, yet the production of the target sound may vary both within and across words.

Virtually all procedures assume that all English sounds should be observed, and in all their potential word positions. While this appears to be a sound decision, there are questions one could raise. First, there is the pragmatic factor of how large a test must be to do this, and the complexity and familiarity of the words needed. Second, some sounds are so infrequent, such as /ʒ/, that it is not clear that its correctness is as important as those with a much higher frequency. Lastly, not even normal children at age six produce all English sounds correctly. We could limit our test words to just those sounds that children have acquired by a certain age, such as four years of age. Shriberg and Kwiatkowski, for example, suggest analyzing the sounds that are in words the child commonly uses, rather than listing every possible sound.

A last point regarding this decision concerns the form of one's phonetic transcription. One issue is whether or not audio taping is done, another is the nature of the transcription. In Ingram (1981), it is suggested that a narrow transcription be used for the permanent record of a child's word, but that a broad one be used for analysis. The broad transcription is less likely to be erroneous, and it allows for the comparison of samples across investigators.

For example, the number of sounds a child is claimed to have will depend upon the fineness of the transcription, with finer transcriptions leading to a larger inventory.

A last decision concerns the practical organization of one's analysis. *Decision 3:* "What is the form of the analysis?" This decision involves aspects such as the forms that record data, the steps in the analysis, and the time it takes to learn and do. In this regard, some specific issues can be considered. For one, are the procedures explicit enough that replication can be done? Articles that provide linguistic analyses of children's data are often so vague that it is unlikely that another analyst would come up with the same results. If an analysis is explicit, there is the further question of the steps to be followed. Some approaches take the analyst through a mysterious maze of steps until suddenly the findings appear. Others, however, can provide insight into the child's language each step of the way. Lastly, one can examine whether the steps of an analysis are flexible or not. For example, if one wants to observe a single feature of the child's system, can that be determined separately, or does the entire analysis need to be done? Decisions on these points can lead to very different analytic procedures, both in terms of the time to learn them and in the information they yield.

Some Problems in Measurement

The single most serious issue facing phonological assessment is that of measurement. Specifically, what is to be measured in deciding that a child does or doesn't have a particular pattern? This is an issue that is often avoided in research in child phonology and one that needs to be resolved before effective assessment procedures are available. Here, I will present seven sets of data samples which demonstrate the kinds of measurement problems that arise.

Data 1: *Syllable vs Word*

[bibo],[ap],[bu],[baba]

[bapi],[bopo],[bopbi],[bapo]

Question: What is the child's system regarding the production of [b] and [p]?

If we use the 'word' as our unit of analysis, we can say that the child uses [b] initially, [p] finally, and both, medially. There is the possibility, however, that the syllable may be the crucial unit. We do not, however, have syllable boundaries marked. It may be, for example, that [b] is syllable initial, and [p] syllable final. If so, we should have our syllables as follows, e.g., [bi-bo], but [bop-o]. Or, we can claim three syllable positions and say that [b] is initial, e.g., [bu] and [bopbi]); [p] is final, e.g., [ap], [bop-bi]; and that they contrast ambisyllabically (between vowels), e.g., [baba][bopo].

The question of syllable boundaries is rarely discussed in works on child phonology. The issue is just as crucial, however, when it comes to substitution analyses. Take, for example, the distinction of /p/ in the following words:

paper, napkin, camping, hope

How do we describe the status of the word internal occurrence of /p/ in "paper," "napkin," and "camping?" The resolution of this requires explicit statements on the use and placement of syllable boundaries (c.f. Ingram, 1981, for some suggestions). Without facing the issue, our analyses will remain incomplete and fuzzy.

Data 2: *Importance of Sample Size*

Child A	[p-]	3×	[b-] 25×	sample size:	150 words
Child B	[p-]	10×	[b-] 10×	sample size:	20 words

Question: What can we conclude by child A's and child B's production of [p] and [b]?

Since both children produce both sounds, we could conclude that both [p] and [b] are acquired. This, in fact, is what most investigators in the past have done. One can challenge this conclusion, however, on the basis of sample size. The child A, for example, has only 3 [p]s out of 150 words, or a 2% occurrence of [p] in the lexicon; [b], on the other hand, is well-established with 17% occurrence. Child B shows a very different picture. Both sounds are dominant and, in fact, constitute all the initial consonants used. Alas, even though child B has less absolute occurrences of [b], its use is greater than that of child A. Data like these indicate that frequency information and sample size are important and necessary for more insight into the child's acquisition of specific speech sounds.

Data 3: *Phonetic Form* vs *Phonetic Type*

Adult Word	Child A	Child B
"Pete"	[pi]	[pit]
"pee"	[pi]	[pi]
"pear"	[pɛ]	[pɛ]
"beer"	[pɛ]	[bɛ]
"me"	[pi]	[mi]

Question: Which child is better at producing [p]?

First, we are examining this question just at the phonetic or articulatory level. If we count words, then A produces [p] five times while B does so only three times. We could conclude from these figures that child A has greater "p" preference. This is only true, however, if we count separate words or *phonetic types*, i.e. distinct phonetic shapes for adult sounds. If we look at *phonetic forms* or unique phonetic shapes, then the opposite picture emerges. Child A has two phonetic forms with [p], [pi], and [pɛ], while child B has three: [pit], [pi] and [pɛ]. With this consideration, child B is now better. We can see that the distinction between phonetic forms and phonetic types is an important one, and that the use of one or the other can lead to different results.

Data 4: *Homonymous Types* vs *Homonymous Forms*

Child A		Child B	
"pat"	[pæt]	"me"	[mi]
"cat"	[pæt]	"knee"	[mi]
"mat"	[pæt]	"coat"	[go]
"tack"	[pæt]	"go"	[go]

Question: Which child has more homonymy?

The above mini-data show four sounds for each child. If one considers each word that is homonymous with another as a homonymous type, then both children have four homonymous types and, therefore, both show equal homonymy. This is not true, however, if we look at homonymous (phonetic) forms. In that case child A has one, [pæt], while child B has two, [mi] and [go]. If we consider a child to be more homonymous based on the number of homonymous types for each homonymous form, then child A is more homonymous since [pæt] occurs for four words. If we choose the number of homonymous forms, however, then child B is more homonymous. Our conclusions are very different, therefore, dependent on what is counted.

Data 5: *What is a substitute?*

"bathtub"	[bætʌ]	/ / → [t]
"balloon"	[bun]	/ / → [b]
"alligator"	[dæge]	/ / → [d]

Question: What sounds do [t], [b], [d] replace in the three words above?

It is rare to see anyone even make explicit how they determine the target sounds for children's substitutions. In many cases, it is easy to see and poses no problems. For example, if the word is "me" and the child says [pi], then [p] replaces /m/. The procedure followed is something like this: line up identical segments between adult and child word, and assume child's nonidentical sounds are substitutions for segments in adult word adjacent to identical segments. There are cases, however, when this is not sufficient, such as the three above. In "bathtub," there are two adjacent segments /θ/, /t/, between the identical vowels. Since the child's [t] is identical to the adult /t/, do we assume that it is a match, or do we consider it as replacing /θ/? In "balloon," our procedure requires us to say [b] has replaced /l/, although we could also argue that [b] matches the adult /b/, and that /l/ has been deleted. Coming up with an explanation of the [d] in "alligator" is particularly challenging, as well as another example of the difficulties of finding appropriate targets. Cases like these show that we need to be more explicit about the ways in which substitutions are determined.

Data 6: *Frequency of Substitutions*

Child A		Child B		Child C	
"car"	[ga]	"car"	[ga] [gæ]	"car"	[ga] [gæ]
"cat"	[gæ]	"cat"	[gæ] [tæ]	"cat" [gæ] [tæ] (5 ×)	
"cake"	[gek]				
"cup"	[tʌ]				

Question: Which child substitutes [g] for /k/ the most?

The issue here is comparable to the one presented by Data 3. For child A, the counts are straightforward: [g] replaces /k/ 75% of the time. For child B, however, some options occur for the calculation. If we count phonetic types, we also get 75%. If we count phonetic forms, however, we get 2 out of 3, or 67%—a lower figure. If we use still another measure, that of percentage of words with the use of a particular sound, then child B has [g] in both words with /k/ for 100%—a higher percentage than child A. Depending on the measure used, child B has less, the same, or more substitutions than child A. This is also true for child C with one further dilemma. If we count phonetic tokens, i.e., any occurrences of a sound, then the five uses of [tæ] will yield a percentage of only 38% for /k/ → [g], since the frequent use of one form can distort this more. Our statements of what a child substitutes depend crucially on the units we choose to count.

Data 7: *What is a Phonological Process?*

Child A	Child B	Child C	Child D
/f/ → [p]	/f/ correct	/f/ correct (3×)	/f/ → [p] 33%
/s/ → [t]	/s/ → [t] 50%	/s/ → [t] (5×)	/s/ → [t] 33%
/ʃ/ → [t,k]	/ʃ/ → [t] 50%	/ʃ/ correct (7×)	/ʃ/ → [t] 33%

The issue of frequency in Data 6 can also be applied to research into phonological processes. Above data are given from four hypothetical subjects on the appearance of the phonological process of Stopping, whereby fricatives are changed into stops. Data like this raise the issue of what is a process, and whether or not we can talk about them independent of individual segments. Child A shows stopping of all fricatives (in data), child D partial stopping of all fricatives, child B stopping of two fricatives, and child C stopping of just one fricative. The data indicate that one cannot just say that a child has a process, but that one must carefully specify what segments are affected and to what degree. It is, in fact, such data which have led researchers to question the predictive value of analyses based on phonological processes.

Some Tentative Answers

My own attempts to face these decisions and questions on measurement are presented in Ingram (1981). Here I will attempt to outline most generally the nature of that work.

Regarding the goal of phonological analysis, I propose four aspects of the child's system that are important to observe: (1) the child's phonetic inventory, (2) the extent of homonymy in the child's words, (3) the kinds of substitutions used for the adult target sounds, and (4) the use of phonological processes. The analysis of a range of behaviours such as these attempts a more complete look at the child's system than many other approaches.

A phonetic analysis examines the sounds used by the child in word initial, medial, and final positions. Unless a child's speech is characterized by one or two striking errors, a phonetic analysis is necessary to get an accurate picture of what the child can and cannot produce. It is also necessary to look at how sounds are produced in different word positions since they may be accurately produced in one position but not in another.

The next three aspects for analysis look at how the child uses the set of sounds produced to represent adult words. One of these aspects is the use of homonymy in the child's output. A young child, for example, might use a phonetic form such as [ba] for two or more adult words, e.g., "bus" and "bottle," creating a pair of homonyms that do not exist in the adult language. Extensive use of homonymy by the child results in low intelligibility and indicates a lack of phonemic proficiency. A homonymy analysis will reveal whether the amount of homonymy in the child's data is normal or excessive.

The substitution analysis shows whether the child's sounds are representing the appropriate adult models or not. For example, if the child produces [f], we need to know if this occurs for the adult /f/, and if it is used as a replacement for other adult sounds, such as /θ/. It is possible to observe children with similar phonetic inventories but different substitution patterns. One child may use his set of sounds mostly for appropriate models, while another child may show widespread substitutions.

If a child does have several substitutions, it is then helpful to pursue a phonological process analysis. Such an analysis pulls together different substitutions into general patterns, which will yield useful information on which substitutions are idiosyncratic and which are the result of a general pattern. The use of this kind of analysis for therapy is discussed by Hodson in this volume.

The second decision concerns the selection of appropriate data for analysis. My preferences are for the kind of sampling suggested in Shriberg & Kwiatkowski (1981). There, the authors recommend the collection of spontaneous utterances from the child, using prompts to elicit a variety of, but not necessarily all, English speech sounds. In the sampling session, it is important to get multiple productions of words so that variability in the child's productions can be observed. Regarding transcription, as mentioned earlier, I use a narrow one for the permanent record, but a broad one for purposes of analysis. The latter lowers one's chance of transcription error and allows comparison to those done by others.

The third decision has to do with the form of one's analysis. One specific aspect of this decision is the explicitness of the approach to analysis. In Ingram (1981), I attempt to deal with this by providing steps to be followed in all analyses. These steps are given in a way that should allow the analyst to come to understand the rationale behind each. Once such understanding is achieved, one can use the steps flexibly, depending on what is to be analyzed. Also, I present various forms that may be used for the recording of one's analysis. A summary of these forms is as follows:

1. Lexicon Sheet: used for recording the phonetic transcription of the child's words.
2. Consonant Inventory Sheets: used for recording the child's productions according to their initial, medial, and final consonants, and also for observing substitutions and calculating their rate of occurrence.
3. Homonymy Sheet: used for recording homonyms and calculating their rate of occurrence.
4. Phonological Process Sheet: used for summarizing the child's phonological processes and calculating their rate of occurrence.
5. Item and Replica Sheet: used for summarizing the child's phonetic inventory and major substitutions.
6. Summary Sheet: used to summarize results from all four analyses.

The use of efficient forms for one's analysis allows for faster analyses and easier retrieval of information.

The most difficult decisions concern the issue of measurement. As pointed out before through seven sets of data, one's choices here will lead to different conclusions about a child's pattern. Data 1 raises the question of syllable versus word position in stating the occurrence of speech sounds. In Ingram (1981), I suggest using the word position for describing the child's phonetic inventory, separating initial, medial, and final positions. This is done because syllable boundaries are rarely marked for child productions, and placement may vary from transcriber to transcriber. For substitution analysis, however, I opt for using syllable boundaries. If a child says [t] for /s/ in "race" and "baseball," for example, both substitutions will be described as a change of /s/ to [t] in syllable final position. To do this, I propose a set of rules to be used in placing syllable boundaries in adult words.

Data sets 2 and 3 both present problems faced in doing a phonetic analysis. To get around problems of sample size, I recommend using a Criterion of Frequency that varies according to sample size. Arbitrarily, I propose that a sound must occur at least once in every 25 words in a sample.

For Data 2, this means that child A must use a sound six times (25 into 150 words) for that sound to be considered used. Thus, [p-] which occurs only three times, is not considered part of the phonetic inventory for child A. This way, one can produce a phonetic inventory for a speech sample that won't be arbitrarily inflated by sample size. Regarding phonetic form versus phonetic type, I propose that phonetic form be used in counting the frequency of a sound. For example, if [pi] represents ten words, it is still only one use of [p-]. This choice requires a sound to occur in diverse phonetic contexts before it is considered frequent. For Data 3, child A uses [p-] twice, i.e., in two phonetic forms, but child B uses it three times, so child B uses [p-] more than child A. This decision combined with the one for Data 2 makes it possible to determine a phonetic inventory for children that is comparable for all analysts.

Data 4 poses problems for one's analysis of homonymy. Above, two measures were presented, one of homonymous lexical types, the other of homonymous phonetic forms. It is not clear to me at this stage of our research which is preferable. To make such a choice will require careful examination of data from several children. In Ingram (1981), both measures are suggested for use until we determine if one is more revealing or representative than the other.

The next two sets of data, 5 and 6, deal with one's substitution analysis. The problem of deciding on the appropriate targets for a child's sounds is a difficult one that is not usually faced by analysts. However, it is possible to set up a list of rules to do this based on natural tendencies in language. Problems arise when consonant clusters are reduced to a single sound, e.g., kl→w. One more commonly finds changes or rules like l→w than k→w. The decision matrix in Ingram (1981, p. 60) proposes to match first on sonorance, then on manner. In kl→w, we say that [w] replaces /l/, rather than /k/, because [w] and [l] both are sonorant sounds. In st→f, all the sounds are obstruents so that this feature cannot be used to make a choice. The next aspect—manner—matches [f] to /s/, since both are fricatives. While decision matrices such as these have a certain degree of arbitrariness, they allow for different analysts to make comparable analyses.

The question of "what to count?" raised by Data 6 for substitution analyses and Data 7 for phonological process analyses is similar to that for phonetic analyses. For substitutions, Ingram (1981) counts one type of substitution per lexical item. For Data 6, child A has three [g] and one [t], child B has two [g] (one for "car" and one for "cat") and one [t], and child C has two [g] and one [t], the same as child B. This decision avoids one highly frequent form such as child C's [tæ] from wrongly giving the impression that [t] dominates the child's productions for /k/. For phonological processes, a conservative line is taken in which calculations of a process are made for each segment affected. The results are presented in terms of (1) which segments are affected by a process, and (2) how extensive is the process for each affected segment. For Data 7, then, all four children show the process of Stopping, but in varying ways.

Concluding Remarks

The three decisions described above and the sample data provided reveal the complex issues involved in attempting to put together an analytic procedure. The sample data are just a selection of the kinds of methodological issues involved in such analyses. I have provided a brief look at attempts to solve these problems as presented in Ingram (1981). The papers in the present volume are representative of alternative approaches and solutions to at least some of these dilemmas. The confrontation with these kinds of problems should constitute a major factor of our efforts in the years ahead, and their resolutions will bring us much closer to efficient and comprehensive analyses and subsequent effective remedial programs.

References

Ingram, D. *Phonological disability in children.* London: Edward Arnold, 1976.

Ingram, D. *Procedures for the phonological analysis of children's language.* Baltimore, Md.: University Park Press, 1981.

Ingram, D., Christensen, L., Veach, S., and Webster, B. The Acquisition of word-initial fricatives and affricates in English by children between 2 and 6 years. In G. Yeni-Komshian, J. Kavanaugh, and C. Ferguson (eds.) *Child Phonology,* vol. 1., 1981.

Shriberg, L., and Kwiatkowski, J. *Natural process analysis, (NPA).* New York: John Wiley, 1980.

Yeni-Komshian, G., Kavanaugh, J., Ferguson, C. (eds.) *Child Phonology,* 2 vols. New York: Academic Press, 1981.

2 Problems Confronting the Theorist and Practitioner in Child Phonology

Joann Fokes

The study of phonological development is of theoretical and practical importance to those in the area of child language study. Presently, there is a vast amount of material on the topic of child phonology. The theorist engages in a search for underlying representation, the determination of natural processes, and the application of rules. Data from the search may support a theory of innate abilities, of physiological maturation, or of dependence upon exposure to the adult system. The intent is the formalization of theories as the result of scientific interest. Theories are based on the analysis and description of data collected from children. Interest in child phonology is also shared by the practitioner who seeks a methodology for an adequate description of children's systems. His/her intent is not theoretical in nature but is in pursuance of matching one child's system against others referred to as normally developing. The intent is the description of a child's system in order to determine its appropriateness. If such a system lacks appropriate features, the practitioner proposes remediation procedures based on normal milestones as speculated by the theorist.

The data at this time are abundant, but diverse in content and in interpretation. Research from different sources leads to conflicting and sometimes confusing conclusions. This is unfortunate, particularly since many practitioners lack sufficient training in phonology to understand the varied findings. Practitioners, quite understandably, are more interested in finding satisfactory methods for analyzing phonological systems and successful procedures for remediation than arguing the specific peculiarities of any one theory.

Regardless of the intent of the investigation, whether theoretical or practical, the investigators need to recognize the necessity for adequate sampling and for appropriate procedures for analysis. The purpose of this paper is not to provide details for procedural analysis, but to point out a number of different problems in variability of speech production that affect sampling and the analysis of child speech. These problems concern both the theorist and the practitioner in the description of phonological systems. Of additional interest to the practitioner is the discussion of remediation procedures for disordered speech. The proposed method is one in which some of the problems encountered in immature and disordered speech can be treated satisfactorily.

Problems in Sampling and Analysis

Each of the following problems has some significance in determining the characteristics of child speech. A failure to understand the effect of each of the problems in variability of production may contribute to confusion in theoretical constructs as well as the mis-diagnosis of a disordered phonological system by the practitioner. It is suggested that each be considered in any attempt at analysis of child speech. A discussion of the following topics will provide some understanding of the apparent variability in child speech. Variability, as described in this paper, is seen at three different levels: (1) variability as a result of different research findings, (2) variability in child pronunciation itself, and (3) variability in procedures for data collection and analysis.

Variability in Research Findings

Findings are reported, and theories are built, on the basis of less-than-adequate data. The procedures for data collection may not be extensive or controlled while the mode of analysis may vary from study to study.

N of 1.   The practitioner is uncomfortable without a mass of data from a large population sample which supports findings in developmental acquisition. Many present-day theories are built on studies of single children, however. Velten (1943), Leopold (1947), Weir (1962), Jakobson (1968), and Smith (1973) contributed large amounts of data, but on single children, and in naturalistic and informal situations. The task, setting, and method were different not only from study to study, but, at times, within the same study. Interestingly, these single subject studies did reveal a number of universal tendencies in acquisition. For example, the vowel distinctions noted by Jakobson were also observed by the other investigators in their children.

Investigations have been limited to single subjects for a number of reasons. Convenience of data collection may have been a factor in the early studies, whereas the extensive amount of time consumption in detailed analysis certainly limited the number of subjects to be investigated. Many studies were carried out over a period of time which contributed greatly to findings in developmental milestones.

Practitioners, who in the past have mistrusted evidence from single-subject studies, may become more accepting of this mode of research once the research problems are recognized. In addition, findings from research may be viewed within a proper perspective and within the limitations of each study. Practitioners must learn to uncover the basic similarities observed from the numerous studies without undue attention to superficial differences among the studies. Practitioners may also learn from the application of data-collection procedures which could be adapted to their own purposes.

Child/Adult Phonology. Many attempts in the analysis of child phonology have followed procedures from the analysis of adult phonology. Waterson (1971) and Menn (1979) argue that child phonology is quite different from any theoretical adult model and should not be based on the adult system. Waterson charges that irregularities occur in the data as the result of analysis procedures based on the adult system.

The practitioner has been more guilty in contriving likenesses and differences of the child system with that of the adult. These descriptions are mostly surface-based, as well. Such a perspective limits a productive methodology being developed in the analysis of child speech.

Presently, there are attempts to include more children in research efforts and to develop models of analysis more adaptable to child speech. Even so, the various ideas put forth by some researchers may cause the practitioner some concern in understanding child phonology.

Variability in Child Speech

Different findings result not only from problems in research design but, also, as the result of variability between groups of children, or within any one child used as a subject for study. Following are some problems to keep in mind in the investigation of child speech.

Phonetic Consistent Forms (PCF). An interesting debate concerns the beginnings of child speech. The question of the importance of babbling as a precursor of speech ranges from the continuity to discontinuity view. Behaviorists claim that selective reinforcement of babbling leads to the development of speech, while others declare there to be no relation between babbling and true speech. The latter feel there are different mechanisms responsible for speech than for vocal play.

As attention has been drawn to the beginnings of speech, especially by psychologists, it has become apparent that infants use vocalizing to communicate during the pre-speech period. Meaningful vocalizations are unlike the babbling noises, yet they are not true words modeled after the adult. Dore, Franklin, Miller, and Ramer (1976) referred to these communicative gestures as Phonetic Consistent Forms. Utterances from time to time were phonetically consistent and served a useful function in the interactional exchange between infants and caretakers. The investigators proposed the

PCFs as a link between the early communicative efforts and the beginnings of true speech.

Ferguson (1978) described similar instances in which early speechlike noises were used with meaning and intent. Although these sounds did not resemble the adult counterpart, the caretaker did respond appropriately. Thus, the "vocables" served a communicative function. The question of the role of these communicative noises is debatable, in that their presence could be an intermediate stage between early communicative efforts and later speech development. The noises may also be explained on the basis of early and immature motor restrictions in sound production.

Following are similar responses heard by this author from Robbie, a late maturing three-year-old:

Phonetic Form	Meaning
[ma:ma]	Do it.
[li:]	Call attention to . . .
[ʔɛʔɛ]	What is it?

The first item was a surprise to the family since the maternal member was missing from the family constellation, and the child had not been exposed to that phonetic sequence. The child used the form when he wanted someone to join him in an activity. The use of this form is interesting in light of the universality of its elements, plus this child's lack of exposure to the sequence. The second sequence was used when he failed, by other means, to apprise others of his play objects. The third form was reserved for requests for names or descriptions of an object. These forms were not used with great frequency but often enough to be recognized as forms with meaning. The infrequent use may have been the result of the child's preference for communicating by other means, such as whining and pointing for needed objects, or head-shaking and withdrawal for rejection of objects or events, such as hand-washing. The forms remained for a period after the occurrence of single words but disappeared as the child slowly gained some conventional control over language.

Since these communication efforts continue well into the speech period, the theorist and the practitioner should recognize their presence, rather than disregarding them as meaningless grunts. A lack of awareness of this phenomenon may cause the investigator to conclude a range of variability of child speech from unintelligible to meaningful.

Idioms and Advanced Forms.   Bloom (1973) and Moskowitz (1980) proposed that the first fifty words were learned as idioms or as independent units. The suggestion is that first words are more pragmatically based than phonologically acquired. It is proposed that the early words arrive outside of the phonological system, although they do aid in carrying out the communicative intents of the child. Some idioms may fairly well match the adult pronunciation as the well-known "pretty" of Leopold's Hildegarde (1947). Her pronunciation at this early stage was referred to as an *advanced form,* in that it better-matched the adult model than her own pronunciation of similar segments in other words. Leopold noted the changes in pronunciation of "pretty" as the child's phonological system progressed. Later pronunciations of "pretty" matched her sound system rather than the adult model. As a result, there appeared to be a regression in her pronunciation of the word when, in fact, it was following the order of her sound system. On the surface, her pronunciation regressed. In actuality, it assimilated into her own sound system. Eventually, her pronunciation once again reached the adult model as her whole segmental system changed to match that of the adult.

Advanced forms or idioms may also be observed in disordered speech, as in the case of Billy, a young boy with a velar preference in pronunciation. Stops and fricatives were velarized with the exception of two advanced forms.

Forms Created from Billy's System		Advanced Forms	
Lexicon	Form	Lexicon	Form
toe	[ko]		
dog	[kɔ]	don't	[do]
daddy	[gagi]	no	[no]
funny	[kʌki]		
Sue	[ku]		
shoe	[ku]		
pencil	[klɪːko]		

Alveolar sounds, particularly, were backed with the exception of two emphatic forms, "don't" and "no." Observation of pronunciation revealed forward placement of the tongue for the two words. These two pronunciations have been maintained and do not match the pattern of pronunciation that is stabilized otherwise. Whether the pronunciation of the two advanced forms is the result of early acquisition or of use of emphatic forms is not known. It is known that these forms presently are outside the child's phonological system.

Idioms may be progressive or regressive in nature. An early-favored pronunciation of a word may be retained for a long period of time after advances have been made in the sound system. As an example, retention of an early pronunciation for suitcase as [hu?kes] was observed by this author for a considerable time after the child had acquired the /s/ in initial position.

The interest of idioms may not supply a great deal of information in the building of theories since the period is brief and the number of observable idioms is generally limited in any one child. Although idioms may not be in abundance in children, the realization of their possible presence may explain apparent variability in child speech. Variability may be the result of use of idioms rather than inherent inconsistency in speech production.

Preferred Forms. Preferred forms differ from advanced forms in that the former are representative of the phonological system while the latter are not. The cautious child may produce only what he is able, or wishes, to attempt. He may refuse to attempt sounds or sound arrangements, particularly multisyllabic sequences or the more difficult sounds such as back stops or fricatives. Although the child may have extensive concepts, he may refuse to pronounce a word that is not consistent with his system. Mothers frequently report that children "know" things or events but will not say them. In some cases, these things may be favored items such as "cookie" or "cake." An example is Sarah, observed by this author, who refused to attempt to say "Keith," although he was her favored sibling in the family. There is the subtle suggestion that children who use preferred forms may be less venturesome than their less cautious counterparts who freely mispronounce forms they have not yet acquired.

An awareness of the use of preferred forms may aid the investigator in the study of child speech in that it provides an explanation of variability among children. Some children may produce many more sound deviations as a result of their willingness to make mistakes or express their thoughts. The less venturesome child will make fewer "errors" in speech, but also express less about his or her environment.

Syllable Structure. Not only are sounds learned early in child phonology, but syllable shapes and sound arrangements are acquired as well. Jakobson (1968) discussed the acquisition of the primary syllable /pa/ by children as their first meaningful word. The syllabic acquisitions coincide with the universals observed as common to the languages of the world. Renfrew (1966) traced syllabic acquisition in the speech-disordered. Her scales included ten stages in the acquisition of the final consonant. Panagos (1974) followed this scale with a scholarly discussion of the linguistic component involved in the failure to acquire final consonants in words. The acquisition of syllabic shape may be viewed as part of linguistic learning. In the early stages, children do tend to omit the final consonant or to reduce the number of syllables in words. Syllable reduction generally occurs on the unstressed syllable in the word or phrase. Ferguson (1978) suggested the notion of a schema for word or phrase-production strategies. Schwartz, Leonard, Wilcox, and Folger (1980) reported findings that reduplication of syllables by children appears to be the result of a strategy for constraining multisyllabic and final consonant production. Klein (1979) probably best described strategies used by some children as either syllable-reducing or syllable-maintaining in the production of multisyllabic words. Children who maintained syllabic configurations frequently were unable to keep phonemic distinctions in their speech while the children who reduced syllables were better able to maintain phonemic distinctions.

A rather extreme case of the effect of syllable structure on pronunciation was observed in Jennifer by this author. This young mentally retarded child had an impressive repertoire of sounds but she produced all words as single open syllables. Below is a list of characteristic pronunciations:

Lexicon	Form	Lexicon	Form
window	[wɪl:]	Sue	[su]
knife	[naɪ]	bus	[bʌ]
fine	[faɪ]	desert	[zɝ·ə]
tree	[ti]	kitty	[kɪi:]
red	[rɛ]	car	[kɔ]
lip	[li]	girl	[gɝ·]
purse	[pɝ·:]	dog	[dɔ]

A brief analysis of the sample shows that intelligibility is virtually absent because of the syllable-reduction processes. The tendency for practitioners to work on sound segments with such children does not bring about improvement in pronunciation.

The product of these findings is that syllable shape plays a role in pronunciation. Apparent variability of segmental production may be due to the segmental arrangement in syllabic configurations. An analysis of child speech should take into account the syllabic conformation as well as the phonetic context resulting from the sound arrangements. Both may have their effect on child speech and bring about variability in production.

Phonetic/Phonemic Differences.   The distinction between phonetic and phonemic abilities is more difficult to distinguish in child phonology than in the adult system. The child's immature physiological system places restrictions upon pronunciation. At first glance, this may appear to be a problem of a phonetic nature. On the other hand, the reported use of idioms in which pronunciation more nearly resembles the adult patterns suggests that children do possess motoric prowess for the articulation of words. In that phonetic proficiency occurs in some instances but not in others is the suggestion that the problem may lie in the establishment of phonemic categories.

The question of the phonetic/phonemic status of segments has been researched also in samples of the omission of the final consonant (Dinnsen, 1980). It has been proposed that the durational aspect of the vowel is suggestive of the status of the final phoneme. Vowel lengthening before the omitted final consonant supplies evidence of the knowledge of the syllable structure of the word, although the final consonant is not produced. A phonetic problem is determined in that instance while the child who does not vary in vowel duration indicates that he lacks knowledge of the presence of final consonants. A phonemic problem is then observed.

The matter is not clear, however, when other examples are provided. In the case of Ryan, as observed by this author, nasals were produced word-initially and intervocalically when a nasal initiated the word as in /mɪni/ for "Minnie" and /no/ for "nose." Production of "pony," "funny," and "penny" were accomplished with an intervocalic flap. An initial analysis suggested the substitution of the nasal with the flap to be of a phonetic nature. Considering the broader scope of phonology beyond a strict segmental basis, one wonders if a phonetic explanation is sufficient when one takes into account the arrangement of segments as part of phonological learning. The use of the flap could be the application of harmony as much as the explanation of a purely phonetic basis.

Although the phonetic/phonemic distinction is a useful concept in descriptive phonology, the breakdown between the two is sometimes difficult to establish in child phonology. It could be that the phases of neuromuscular and physiological growth are quite interrelated and intertwined with cognitive and linguistic development. Growth in both areas may lead to the establishment of phonological distinctions. Learning to control the arrangement of segments could be a part of phonological development.

Early Oppositions/Contrasts.

A cornerstone in developmental phonology is the concept of phonemic opposition. Sounds in words are contrastive with each other on the basis of bringing about a change in meaning. The issue of contrastiveness was formally presented by Jakobson (1968) and modified and expanded by Menyuk (1968), Moskowitz (1970), and Blache (1981). Jakobson's explanation of the development of contrasts is based on the presence of linguistic universals in language. In addition, diary studies which report instances of contrasts suggest that their acquisition is brought about by pragmatic necessity or the need to be understood.

While later writings do not verify feature acquisition to the extent Jakobson outlined, there is still the suggestion that feature acquisition occurs in an orderly manner. Jakobson failed to take into account phonetic context in his model, which affects the production of sound contrasts. For those interested in the analysis of child speech, it is suggested that context-free segment arrangements be set up for obtaining samples as well as various phonetic contexts in evaluating the presence of contrasts in child speech. The investigator may, in fact, observe variability in child speech as the result of the variation in the context offered. For example, contrasts may be observed more easily in List 1 than in List 2, in which the phonetic environment of the final sound may affect the contrast.

Alveolar/Velar Contrast

List 1	List 2
tea/key	tight/kite
dough/go	date/gate
day/gay	tape/cape
two/coo	tick/kick

The context-free condition of List 1 may allow for contrasts if, indeed, they are present. The final sounds, particularly when the same as one of the members of the contrast, may affect the production of the contrast. If context is used, the third pair of List 2 would be preferred since the final member is not the same as that of the contrasts, although there are feature similarities.

Stress.   Wieman (1976) found the use of stress patterns in children below the age of two years. Stress is known to affect adult pronunciation and, quite possibly, may affect children's. The amount of stress given to a word is dependent upon its role within the sentence and the intention expressed. Words are affected by any number of reduction procedures. Changes may occur in production of stressed syllables, in that attention is directed toward the pragmatic effect of the word rather than precise production. Perhaps the less-stressed syllables may match the adult production when the pragmatic load is reduced. Unstressed syllables may be affected by any number of reduction procedures.

Variability of sound production may be observed in changes of stress brought about by differing pragmatic intents. Investigators should observe the extent of variability in production as the result of stress.

Perception.   At present, linguists are hesitant to draw relations between the information in perceptual studies and those of production. Most theorists acknowledge that perception precedes production, but few attempt to develop a theory of production as dependent or related to perception. An exception is Waterson's (1971) theory. Her analysis of child data pronunciation was explained on the basis of the effect of the child's perceptual schemata of speech. By her reasoning, perception occurs globally and is transferred to pronunciation in a similar manner, rather than in a segmentally ordered manner. As an example, nasality may be perceived and produced, but its production may not occur in the matched segment of the adult pronunciation. The child's ability to produce words is based on the perceptual schemata of word configurations. Perception and production are affected by the structural scheme present in the child's system.

Other perceptual studies have not directly linked the perception of speech to production, but have looked at perception itself. Many of the perceptual studies summarized by Morse (1978) demonstrated that infants are capable of making auditory discriminations between speech sounds, at least physiologically. There is some debate about whether phonemic processing takes place at this early age or if the skill is attributed to the infants' physiological ability.

Other perceptual studies by Shvachkin (1973) and Barton (1978) have employed older infants and young children. Young children are able to make phonemic distinctions at an early age according to the findings. Phonemic distinctions are dependent upon word knowledge, however.

The effect of perception on production is not clear but, certainly, investigators should take perceptual skills into account in the analysis of speech samples. Variability in productions may occur as the result of different structural schemata affecting word production.

Homonymy.   Ingram (1977) has stated that homonymy is one of the important factors in child speech as well as in disordered speech. Children with an excessive number of homonyms are unable to make themselves understood. Homonyms are brought about by a lack of contrast of phonetic segments or problems in syllable configuration. If syllable reduction or reduplication takes place, the child is unable to produce the needed distinctions in order to be understood. Homonyms could be created by any one, or combination, of the problems discussed so far. As in the case of Billy, who was previously discussed, his speech was characterized by numerous homonyms based on lack of contrasts as well as syllable reduction processes. Examples include the following:

Lexical Contrasts	Phonetic Representation
pea/tea/Dee/tree/street	[ki]
pie/prize/tie/dry/sky	[kaɪ]
Pooh/two/true/drew/screw	[ku]
fine/pine/time/dime/pie/tie	[kaɪ]
pencil/pedal/nickle/Christmas	[kiku]

Homonymy becomes even more interesting in the case of Billy, who was able to make perceptual contrasts quite easily and who severely objected to some of his pronunciations when repeated to him. The relation between perception and production becomes a significant question. It is of greater importance in that Billy was a constant chatterer who freely used homonyms in communication. Interestingly, Priestly (1980) and Vihman (1979) have shed some light on the problem.

Priestly (1980) has described different types of homonymy. He refers to true homonymy in which there are no articulatory or perceptual contrasts. In some instances of homonymy, the child may be making contrasts that are not discernible to the listener. Priestly contends that there is an important distinction between true homonymy and the other types, and that they should be identified.

Vihman (1979) proposed that homonymy may be used as a strategy by some children for production of words. These children lack control of phonemic contrasts and may resort to homonymy in order to express what it is that he knows about his world.

Motivation to Change.   Some children seem to be sensitive to adult phonology and attempt to match it, while others are quite satisfied with their own efforts to be understood. The latter do little to modify their speech pattern. Others may attempt to change, but are not able to proceed through the developmental stages. These children may be confronted with frustration in their inability to be understood. The practitioner should be sensitive to this factor in testing and remediation.

Change as the Result of Emerging Stages. One of the observations of child speech is that it is not static, but changing, in a path toward adult pronunciation. The child's speech at any one time may be represented by its current stage, remnants of a preceding stage, and emergence from a succeeding stage. Practically, this is the desired state of affairs. In data collection, the three stages may be represented in samples. Since the stages are defined by differences in articulation, there may be differences as the three stages interfere with one another. There may be interference from the preceding and succeeding stages, which also brings about a degree of variability in child speech. Perhaps the three different levels can be recognized in the sample. The resulting variability on the surface can be seen as change, rather than inconsistency, in child speech.

Summary. Many problems have been discussed which would bring about differences in speech production among children and within the individual child. On the surface, some of the resulting data would suggest that there is a great deal of variability among children in the acquisition of their native language, and that common milestones are not present. In understanding the various problems as discussed, one is able to search below surface pronunciation and determine commonalities. In addition, these problems may cause a great deal of irregularity in an individual child, rendering production differences from one attempt to another. Again, in understanding problems confronting the immature speaker and the disordered speaker, one is able to understand the apparent irregularities and determine the commonalities.

Variability in Data Collection Procedures

Several methodologies are presently available which provide instructions for data collection and for the sampling of individual speech problems. These methodologies contain specific guidelines for data collection and offer arguments for specific points to be covered in the collection procedure. The following discussion addresses some problems concerning these data collection procedures.

Citation/Context. Most investigations point out the superiority of obtaining examples in context form as opposed to citation form in order to get a more natural form of speech. Rather than arguing about the advantages of one method over the other, it is suggested that both forms should be used in obtaining samples of speech. A comparison of both forms will provide a measure of variability between the two productions. Among some speech-disordered children, citation does not always provide the better-produced form in that context supplies support for the speaker as well as the listener. Some productions could be judged more acceptable in conversation form than in citation with the support of the context. In other instances, citation may be the situation in which the child can render the most acceptable effort since the speaking load is reduced.

The merits of citation form become apparent in instances in which children are extremely limited in vocal output and cannot tolerate a contextual testing situation. This form may seem to be the child's best effort in some cases. Certainly the investigator would want to have representations of both forms of speech. It should be pointed out that contextual testing is most effective when a target word is embedded within a phrase or sentence. If the target word is the last word of the phrase or sentence, its production is similar to citation form in that there is no outside boundary. In this writer's experience, testing in context with the target word at the end of context is not satisfactory because children frequently lack sufficient air-control to produce the word audibly and satisfactorily.

Spontaneous/Imitated Forms. The most desirable form, according to many investigators, is a spontaneously collected speech sample which is a better representation of natural speech. Imitated forms sometimes are better-produced because of modeling. The child may be able to change his natural response when given a model to imitate. There are, however, some children who cannot imitate successfully. Their imitations are noticeably inferior to their spontaneous speech. Perhaps the pragmatic value of the imitated form is so low that it does not warrant a reasonable attempt from the child. The effect of a memory factor should also be considered. Just what mechanisms are operating or what mechanisms are failing at this time is up to speculation. In that imitated forms are thought to be superior because of the modeling effect, a failure to benefit from modeling is certainly an item of interest and should be taken into account in the assessment period.

The use of imitated forms in assessment has been shoved to a secondary place since spontaneous speech is the more natural form. Imitated forms are generally reserved for instances in which the investigator is unable to obtain a spontaneous sample. The suggestion here is that word, phrase, and sentence imitation is known to have prognostic value as far as the ability to effect change with a model. On this basis, it has value in the testing procedure. In addition, there are those children who just cannot imitate and do not profit from the model. Certainly these should be identified, and appropriate remediation procedures should be planned on the basis of this inability.

The debate of the use of spontaneous or imitated sampling brings to mind the *trade-off* phenomenon as defined by Garnica and Edwards (1976). While imitated and repeated productions were thought to bring about improvements in pronunciation, Garnica and Edwards found that there were segmental changes within the productions rather than overall improvement. That is, if, in the initial effort, a segment was off target in pronunciation, the segment may be improved with imitation and repetition. Other segments of the original production, however, were modified to the extent that the target pronunciation was not maintained. The authors noted what they called a *trade-off* in which original segments were modified in succeeding repetitions.

Some segments, originally correct, become incorrect—while original incorrect segments became correct. This study, as much as any other work, points out the variability in child speech. Certainly the extent and degree of variability should be noted in studies of child language.

Repair.   In conversation, there may be breakdowns of communication because of speech intelligibility. When this occurs, a request for a repair may be made. The speaker may be asked to repeat his production in order that the conversation continue. One of the most elementary forms of repair is a phonetic change from the original production. Thus, when children are asked for a repetition of what they have said, their response may be altered from the original meaning, in that they attempt a more precise articulation. The change of articulation suggests their awareness of the inadequacy of the first attempt and the resulting effort toward greater precision. Phonetic change, however, can be both progressive and regressive in nature. That is, a progressive change is one in which the original utterance may miss target production but be improved in the repair, while the reverse takes place for a regressive change. If this is true, some repairs may be better characterized by inherent variability rather than pragmatic effort.

Children may be aware of the pragmatic nature of requests for repair. They may process a request for a repetition in a test situation as a request for a repair. In satisfying the listener, they may attempt a greater level of precision by altering the original production. On the other hand, change in the articulatory effort may not be motivated by any effort toward precision, but it may be the result of the child's natural tendency of variability. That is, the child's system may be so unstable that a phonetic change is effected regardless of the pragmatic knowledge. The use of a repair technique in requesting repetitions may be effective in data collection procedures. The investigator will have the opportunity to view whether or not a change takes place, and if it does, the degree and direction to which the original effort is repaired.

Task.   Most investigators are well aware that the degree of success in data collection is dependent upon the task level and interest, as well as the child's understanding of it. In addition, it should be pointed out that the task should be suited to the intent of the investigator in obtaining the type of sample desired.

Summary.   The preceding discussion referred to aspects or problems that confront the investigator in collecting speech samples. Although time limitations may prohibit extensive testing and the use of different procedures, the advantages of using speech samples obtained by citation and contextual form, imitated and spontaneous speech, and the use of a repair-type approach should be considered. In addition, the task, as well as the child's understanding of the task, are crucial to the sample collection.

While the theorist and the practitioner are both interested in data collection, the theorist probably does not share the practitioner's concern for any type of remediation procedure. The theorist is interested in the description of the system of child phonology and its relation to that of adult phonology. Theorists are now involved in the description of deviant speech, an interest shared with the practitioner. The practitioner, however, must take the data and plan remediation procedures based upon findings from the analysis. Following is a suggestion for remediation procedures that takes into account some of the problems noted in child study.

Application of Phonemic Contrasting as a Remediation Procedure

Phonemic contrasting is a concept familiar in linguistics and used in the process of the discovery of phonemic systems. Sounds in a language differ from one another on the basis of a set of features that can be described in articulatory terms or, if desired, in acoustic terms. Certain sounds may vary in several dimensions. Those that are called minimal pairs vary minimally from one another (i.e., by only one feature) while others may vary in several dimensions. Linguists are able to categorize sound systems of languages on the basis of testing for minimal pairs. If two sounds, each found in the same phonetic context, change the meaning of a word, then both sounds possess phonemic status in the language. For instance, "tea" and "key" vary by one feature of place of articulation in the mouth. The /t/ in "tea" and the /k/ in "key" possess similar articulatory features, with the exception of the place of articulation. A change of this one feature results in the change of the phoneme which, in turn, changes the meaning of the word. The feature causing the change is distinctive in nature in that it brings about the change in meaning. Other pairs of sounds may vary by more than a single feature. For instance, the /s/ in "see" varies from the /k/ in "key" by several features.

Jacobson (1968) used phonemic or feature contrasts in his writings about child acquisition of language. His descriptions traced development of the sound system on the basis of feature acquisition rather than segmental learning. Although child sound acquisition has not been found to be as systematic as he described, the concept of phonemic contrasts is a useful one in the study of child phonology. It may also be used with individuals with speech disorders in that its procedures can deal with the problems noted in this paper. Phonemic contrasting can be applied as a therapeutic aid in acquiring contrasts. It should be pointed out that the procedures are therapeutically devised rather than based on a strict developmental scheme. A brief explanation of the Phonemic Contrasting methodology follows.

The Phonemic Contrasting Methodology

The method is a simple one to apply and can bring about changes in disordered systems in several dimensions. A few materials are required, a systematic procedural approach is needed, and a scoring procedure should be used.

Materials: Picture cards are needed to represent words or events. The pictured word cards are arranged in pairs. The two words that make up the pair are words that vary on the basis of particular features. For instance, a picture of "tea" and a picture of "key" may be used to represent a "tongue-front/tongue-back" contrast. Several picture-word cards representing the contrast should be made.

A Phonemic Contrasting Board is also useful as a device for calling attention to the phonemic contrast represented by the word pairs. Labels, drawings, or schematic representations of the contrast may be placed on the board. The therapeutic display should define the characteristics of the opposing members of the pair.

A scoring sheet for marking the individual's progress should be developed.

Procedure: Procedures for phonemic contrasting may vary considerably as demanded by the nature of the individual problem. The following are suggested procedures that may be applied:

1.   Select eight to ten pairs of word cards that represent the contrast to be presented. Place the cards on the Phonemic Contrasting Board below the drawing on the board that defines the contrast. Separate the cards into the two opposing decks. Examples of word lists are the following pairs for four different contrasts. Note that the word pairs do not necessarily have to be minimal but should represent the contrast under study.

Alveolar/Velar	Open/Closed	Mono/Bisyllabic	Breaking Up Assimilation
Dee/key	pie/pipe	pop/poppy	tot/top
tar/car	row/road	Bub/bubble	cock/cop
tear/care	bye/bike	cook/cookie	tight/kite
two/goo	sew/soap	pick/pickle	boom/boot
dust/gust	pea/peak	pay/paper	peep/peak

2.   The teacher pronounces each of the words and places each word in a context. The word pairs are also to be identified according to the articulatory oppositions presented. The word card is then placed on

the Phonemic Contrasting Board by the label or drawing which defines the contrast. The child identifies the word card as the teacher pronounces.

3. The child then attempts the contrast. If the contrast is not achieved, the teacher asks for a repair. If needed, the teacher may cue the child as to the desired articulatory gesture in order to bring about more acceptable pronunciation.

4. The child's response is scored, not in terms of correct pronunciation of the whole word, but in terms of whether or not the contrast was achieved.

5. Rather than extensive drill on a word pair, the next word pair is presented in a similar fashion. If allowed, most children engage in practice of a word pair and use the word in context similar to the model given by the teacher.

6. From time to time, the child may match the word card with the appropriate display on the Phonemic Contrasting Board.

7. The teacher may ask for pronunciations from the child without models. In doing so, the teacher would identify the child's pronunciation by pointing to the picture card that illustrated what the child had articulated. For instance, if the child intended to say "key" but said "tea," the teacher would point to the picture of "tea" indicating to the child a need for a change in the articulatory pattern.

8. After the word pairs have been presented, the decks may be presented again in a similar fashion. With each representation, the teacher asks for additional contextual information in conjunction with the pronunciation of the word pairs.

9. The session may terminate with the use of as many of the word pairs as possible in an on-the-spot, made-up story context. The story should relate to the child's interest as much as possible.

10. Work on the contrast continues until the teacher is satisfied that the child has acquired the distinction.

The following is a dialogue recorded between a clinician and a hearing-impaired client who backed alveolar sounds. The contrast presented was the alveolar/velar contrast. Voicing and other contrasts or pronunciations were not emphasized at this time.

The clinician presented the appropriate
pictures as the session progressed.

Child	Clinician
	Child picks up a picture
	Yes, a car. And this is a picture of tar. The tar is gooey, and the tar is on the car. Remember to move your tongue to the front of your mouth and say "tar."
/ka:/	
	What did you say? Did you say "car?" Say "tar."
/ta:/	
/ta:/, . . ./ka:/	Yes, tar. Tar is on the car.
	Now, here is Dee. She has a key to the car. What does she have?
/ki/	
	A key. Who has the key?
/ki/	
	Who? Not "key" but "Dee." Move your tongue to the front of your mouth. Say "Dee."
/di/ /di/ have a /ki/. a /ki/ in the /ka:/	
	And what does the car have on it?
/ka:/ have /ka:/	
	The car has what?
/ta:/ on /ka:/	

The clinician presents all word pairs
in a similar manner until the deck
of words is completed.

Child	Clinician
	Now, let's tell our story. This is a story about Dee. Dee has a key to a car. Dee has a key.
/di/ have /ki/	
	Dee is riding down the road in her car. The road is full of tar. Tar is on her car.
/ka:/ on /ka:/	
	What? What is on the car? Tar?
/ta:/ is on the /ka:/	

.... /gʌ/ of wind. It blow ..... /dʌ/.

A gust of wind blew on the car. Now the car is full of dust. A gust of wind blew dust on the car.

/kʊ:/ point to . . . /dʊ:/. /ka:/ have /ta:/, too.

/ka:/ /gui/, /tu/.

Dee saw Kurt down the road. Kurt said, "Look at the dirt on the car." Kurt pointed to the dirt.

Yes, it full of goo, too. It's gooey.

Dee said, "I must take care of my car. I don't want to tear up my car. I don't want to . . ."

......

/tɛə/ up, /tɛə/ up car.

I don't want to tear up my car.

/ke ke/

Yes, Dee wants to take care of her car.

/te ke, te ke/

Take care.

/te ke/ of /ka:/

Take care of the car.

/gi/

Who? Who is taking care of the car?

.... /gi/ . . . /di/

Who? What's her name?

Yes, Dee. Dee has a car. And Dee has a key.

Advantages in the Use of Phonemic Contrasting

Phonemic contrasting is a reasonable approach to remediation in that it provides the procedures for designating contrast in speech. Since a major problem of disordered speech is lack of contrasts, this method is particularly helpful in that the oppositions in speech are emphasized. The child becomes aware of the contrasts on a semantic, as well as an articulatory, basis. The contrasts are defined in terms of the difference in meaning of words and that a sound brings about the difference. If the child does not produce a sound distinction in the word pairs, he is exposed to the resulting confusion between the words. He may also experience some pragmatic problems as a consequence of the confusions. The child then puts forth the effort to change articulatory gestures in order to clear up the semantic confusions. With the acquisition of contrasts, homonymy and preferred forms may be reduced in child speech. With the realization of the distinction of sounds in words, the degree and extent of variability in repeated productions will be reduced.

The procedures avoid some of the problems that may create variability in child speech in that pure drill is not carried out. Word cards are presented for the child's production, but numerous repetitions are not requested. Instead the child "practices" by repeating in a more natural manner. In addition, the use of context supplies a reason for explicitness in pronunciation. The child finds that he enjoys supplying his own context.

A variety of problems may be attacked through phonemic contrasting. Any type of contrast may be presented and not simply minimally paired contrasts. The choice of contrasts depends upon the nature of the problem observed in the speech pattern. If the child's system contains few sounds, maximal contrasts may be initiated in order to establish major categories. These may not necessarily match the adult system, but they may be more appropriate to the stage into which the child is evolving.

Phonemic contrasts may be presented by comparing word pairs with sound differences in the initial position of words. In severe cases, this type of contrast is suggested in open-syllable words in order that phonetic context does not affect pronunciation of the contrasts. In other instances, the contrasts may be placed in the final position of words. Contrasts may represent any type of articulatory gesture, such as place of articulation, difference in voice-onset time, or differences in the manner of articulation. Not only can consonant contrasts be taught, but vowel contrasts may be presented, as well. Consonant singletons may be contrasted with clusters. This type of contrast also employs a difference in the shape of the words contrasted. Thus, phonemic contrasting may also be used to train various syllable shapes. For instance, the open syllable can be quite easily contrasted with a variety of closed-syllable words for children who have syllable-structure problems. Single-syllable words may also be contrasted with bisyllabic words. In fact, the procedures can be planned to break down many of the possible strategies found in immature and disordered speech.

Another advantage to the methodology is that more than a single contrast can be presented during a session. It is suggested, however, that if several contrasts are presented in a session, they be presented one at a time in order to eliminate any confusion as to the articulatory gesture requested.

The method can be used individually or with small groups of children. Small groups work well in that they facilitate observance of other children's pronunciation efforts. The method has application to a variety of disordered speech cases, ranging from structural and organic problems to those with no apparent cause. The semantic and pragmatic basis of the method appear to reinforce the idea of contrastiveness even though mechanical problems impede the ability to produce speech. In doing so, variability as reported in child speech may be reduced.

Summary

Several problems confronting the theorist and practitioner in child phonology were pointed out in this discussion. Problems in methodology include results based on single-subject diary studies and the application of adult models to child study. Some of the information is not only diverse and unrelated, but conflicting in nature. Many of the conflicting results appear as descriptions of single children rather than attempts toward uncovering the generalities of the findings.

The problems encountered in child speech itself make it difficult to study. A recognition of the problems will aid in collections of data as well as in the interpretation of the findings. Researchers will find it necessary to differentiate between linguistic forms and forms that are not linguistically derived, but perhaps more pragmatically derived. Such forms include the early communication efforts that are functional in child speech but dissimilar to the phonetic forms used in the adult language. Prelinguistic forms, such as phonetic consistent forms or vocables, as well as idioms or advanced forms, should be considered outside the emerging phonological system.

The realization that children appear to place restrictions on themselves in their speech, in a manner of speaking, will aid in understanding some of their questionable behavior. Some children are quite exploratory in the use of new forms to express themselves, while others are more cautious. The latter may refuse to attempt new forms although they may be quite knowledgeable about their world. These children may use only preferred forms to express what they know.

The developing system is subject to a number of restrictions in syllable structure and contrastiveness in segmental forms. The path of acquisition of syllable structure and feature contrasts is not clearly marked if observed on the surface only. Children may vary in strategies in the acquisition of the forms required for the sound system, although there may be commonalities in the processes used. Attempts to explain restrictions have been made on both phonetic and phonemic bases. Considering the motor limitations and cognitive stage and the interaction of these two areas of growth, this author finds it difficult to make clearly marked distinctions between phonetic and phonemic problems. A realization of the close relationship between the two is suggested.

A particularly interesting area of study is that of perception and its influence on production. Its role in the developing system should be considered.

The problems noted may cause one of the outstanding characteristics of early child speech—that of homonymy. With the restricted syllable and segmental distinctions, a great number of homonyms are heard in child speech. One must be aware of the processes that bring about the similarities in production. These same processes may, however, be the cause of the degree of instability observed in child speech as well.

The problems may be considered in their own light, but they take place in the setting of an emergent system. Any problem noted herein is imposed upon a system that is subject to some type of maturational or developmental change. The emergent system would seem to bring about fluctuation in the system in interaction with the problems noted. While this may cause concern enough, one must remember that the disordered system is one that is slow to effect change. Although unstable in many aspects, the speech-and language-disordered are those who remain in immature stages for prolonged periods. It is with this population that many practitioners wish to bring about change.

The method suggested to effect change is phonemic contrasting. The purpose of the method is to bring about the realization of contrast in syllable structure and in segmentals in words and phrases. The realization may be presented on the basis of changes in articulatory differences, but the method relies on the semantic differences that cause the need for articulatory adjustments. The goal may be pragmatic in nature, or the need to be more precise and explicit in communication. While the language components may be satisfied through the use of techniques to specify the need for articulatory adjustments, practice in a functional way is also provided. In fact, with creative use of the method, the child becomes his own guide in practice. He makes his own repeated attempts to be understood. Many of the problems of early speech and disordered speech, one hopes, may be replaced by the rules descriptive of the adult system.

References

Barton, David. *The Role of Perception in the Acquisition of Phonology.* Bloomington, Ind.: University Linguistics Club, 1978.

Blache, Stephen. (This volume, 1981)

Bloom, Lois. *One Word at a Time,* The Hague: Mouton, 1973.

Dinnsen, D. Paper Presentation at Midwest Child Phonology Society. Champaign-Urbana, Illinois, 1980.

Dore, John, Franklin, M.B., Miller, R.T., and Ramer, A.L. Transitional phenomenon in early language acquisition, *Journal of Child Language,* 1976, *3,* 13–28.

Ferguson, C.A. Learning to pronounce: the earliest stages of phonological development in the child. *Communicative and Cognitive Abilities,* Minifie, F.D. and Lloyd, L.L. (eds.), Baltimore: University Park Press, 1978.

Garnica, Olga and Edwards, Mary Louise. Phonological variation in children's speech: the trade-off phenomenon. *Ohio State Working Papers,* 1977, *22,* 81–87.

Ingram, David. *Phonological Disability in Children,* New York: Elsevier, 1977.

Jakobson, Roman. *Child Language, Aphasia, and Phonological Universals,* The Hague: Mouton, 1968.

Klein, Harriet. The relationships between perceptual strategies and productive strategies in learning the phonology of early lexical items. Dissertation, Brooklyn College, 1978. (Available from Indiana University Linguistics Club, Bloomington, Indiana.)

Leopold, W.F. *Speech Development of a Bilingual Child,* Vol. II, Chicago: Northwestern University Press, 1947.

Menn, Lise. Towards a Psychology of Phonology: Child Phonology as a First Step. Conference Proceedings, Michigan State University, 1979.

Menyuk, Paula. The role of distinctive features in children's acquisition of phonology. *Journal of Speech and Hearing Research,* 1968, *11,* 138–146.

Morse, Phillip A. Infant speech perception: origins of processes, and alpha centauri. *Communicative and Cognitive Abilities,* Minifie, F.D. and Lloyd, L.L. (eds.), Baltimore: University Park Press, 1978.

Moskowitz, B. Arlene. The two-year-old stage in the acquisition of English phonology, *Language,* 1970, *46,* 426–441.

Moskowitz, B. Arlene. Idioms in phonology acquisition and phonological change. *Journal of Phonetics,* 1980, *8,* 69–83.

Panagos, John. Persistence of the open syllable reinterpreted as a symptom of language disorder, *Journal of Speech and Hearing Disorders,* 1974, *39,* 23–31.

Priestly, Tom M.S. Homonymy in child phonology, *Journal of Child Language,* 1980, *7,* 413–427.

Renfrew, Catherine, E. Persistence of the open syllable in defective articulation, *Journal of Speech and Hearing Disorders,* 1966, *31.*

Schwartz, Richard, Leonard, Laurence, Wilcox, M. Jeanne, and Folger, M. Karen. Again and again: reduplication in child phonology. *Journal of Child Language,* 1980, *7,* 75–87.

Shvachkin, N.K. The development of phonemic speech perception in early childhood. *Studies of Child Language Development,* Ferguson, C.A. and Slobin, D. (eds), New York: Holt, Rinehart, and Winston, 1973.

Smith, N. *The Acquisition of Phonology: A Case Study.* Cambridge: Cambridge University Press, 1973.

Velten, H. The growth of phonemic and lexical patterns in infant language. *Language,* 1943, *19,* 281–292.

Vihman, M.M. Phonology and the Development of the Lexicon. Department of Linguistics, Stanford University, 1979.

Waterson, N. Child phonology: a prosodic view. *Journal of Linguistics,* 1971, *7,* 170–221.

Weir, Ruth. *Language in the Crib,* The Hague: Mouton, 1962.

Wieman, Leslie. Stress patterns of early child language. *Journal of Child Language,* 1976, *3,* 283–287.

3 Diagnostic Assessment of Developmental Phonological Disorders

Lawrence D. Shriberg

The Rhotacist and the Maytag Repair Man

Those of us with a long-standing interest in phonology have reason to be happy about this collection of papers. Phonological disorders seem to have come of age. Until just a few years ago, in fact, I suspect that most of the contributors to this volume had to be content with wearing only one of two hats.

One hat I have worn a lot since beginning to teach at a university is the hat of a "rhotacist." I am indebted to John Locke for this Lockian play on words. John suggested that since the /r/ is a rhotic sound, /r/ specialists might appropriately be called "rhotacists." I rather like the term. The rhotacist's particular domain, of course, is the "tough /r/ kid" (Shriberg, 1975; 1980). When a school speech pathologist has become desperate about a tough /r/ kid, a child who simply can't seem to say a good /r/, the one last chilling possibility is to " . . . call in THE RHOTACIST." And, from the speech and hearing department of the local university comes the rhotacist with his or her bag of tricks to drive out the evil /r/ distortion and evoke a good and pure /r/. Calls for a rhotacist have been frequent, year after year. My rhotacist hat is well-worn, and I'm comfortable with it.

Like the Maytag repair man, however, during the early 1970s I did not have many calls to see children with severely delayed speech. In fact, only recently have I been able to properly break in my repair-man hat. Why? Certainly, the interest in language disorders that swept the field during the late 1960s and 1970s should have embraced children with phonological disorders. Certainly, children with severely delayed speech development qualify as having both a disability and a handicap, and hence, meet state and federal requirements for receiving special school services. Yet, I spent much of the early 70s waiting for calls that never came.

I think one important reason for the lack of clinician-level interest in children with developmental phonological disorders could be traced to the type of literature published in the 70s. Many different approaches to phonological assessment have appeared. Speech pathologists have been faced with the task of deciding whether any of these new materials are really relevant to clinical practice. Clinicians who have attempted to follow this literature may not be convinced that emerging procedures offer truly new and helpful management possibilities. Why should one take the time to learn new terms and learn to administer and score lengthy measures if the results are only a page full of percentages that are not really telling?

To end these few observations, I note that only very recently have calls routinely come in to assess and suggest ways to "repair" children with more severe phonological disorders. To enrich methodological procedures in "functional articulation disorders" (Bankson, 1980), we must add substance, not simply alternative tallying schemes. I look forward to the continuing dialogue.

Case Example

What kinds of calls do come in for children with more severe phonological involvement?

Dan is a 5½–year–old boy referred to us for assistance in assessing his disorder and in developing a management plan for his severely delayed speech development. A gloss and transcription of 20 utterances of his speech is presented in Figure 1. Does his speech pattern look similar to that of other children you have seen? What is his problem? Can you tell from this sample (1) why Dan has delayed speech? (2) how severely involved is his speech? (3) when, if ever, he will self-correct his errors? (4) which type of currently available management approach, if any, should be tried with him? These are the questions we are expected to answer in a diagnostic appraisal. Can you answer them on the basis of the information presented in Figure 1? If not, what other information would you require?

The point of this opening example is the very point of my presentation. I think that it is time that we become seriously concerned with *diagnostic assessment*. Specifically, I think that our research and clinical procedures must be focused on etiological differences among children who present delayed speech acquisition. I suggest that a truly systematic account of the origins of speech delay and the implications for management that follow can be gained only from differential diagnostic studies. Until we begin to relate phonological description to physiological and psychological data on the person whose behavior is being described, I think we will continue to generate only more numbers. And I simply do not think that more description will lead us out into the light. Before continuing with some possible answers to the questions posed about Dan, let us look briefly at some theoretical issues that form the background for our work.

child Dan DOB 9-24-74

Age 5-2

Sampling 12-12-79 Analysis _____

Date _____ Date 1-24-80

Clinician _____

NPA TRANSCRIPTION SHEET

Shriberg and Kwiatkowski
John Wiley & Sons   Copyright 1980 NPA

Comments on _____

Sample _____

Conditions _____

Item No.	GLOSS	TRANSCRIPTION	Item No.	GLOSS	TRANSCRIPTION
	We got playdough at home. Yeah.	du ʔə 'bēɪjo ʔɛʔ ʔõʊ jɛʌ		Her got more play-dough for me an. Julie.	ɝ at ɛ̄ɪ 'mofə beɪo o mi ŋ dʒuːi
➤	At Julie. Yeah.	ət 'dʒuːwēɪʰ jɛ̄		My mom throw away Julie playdough.	māɪ mã oʊ əweɪ dʒuːwi 'bēɪdo
	My sister. Um hum.	māɪ 'jæʔ̃ mhm̩		and her got me some more playdough.	ɛ̄ ɜ ʔəʔ mi ə mɔʊ 'bēɪjo
	Her eight. Yep.	ʔɜ ʔēɪ jɛpʔ		a bear	'bēɪjə
	An xx x xx x	ɛ̃n 'ılõ mɔɪ ʌ̃nõ 'uː		I did bear. Right there. Yeah	ʌ̃ dɪd bēɪɜ raɪʔ dɛʌ jɛʌ
	Her little brother	ʔɜ ĩwə 'bʌʔə		Button. There elephant.	bʌʔn̩ dɛʔ 'ɛːʌẽʔ
	x x x xx	ēɪʔ ĩm ə 'ēɪja		and flower an' a flower	ɛ̃nd 'ʔaʊɜ ɛ̃n ə 'ʔaʊə
	x xx x	māɪ ʌ̃ndwɛ̃ʔ ʔju		an' a um	ɛ̃n ə ʌ̃m
	x xx xx	ēɪ ʔəwõ ēɪjʌʰ		yeah, what are these? xx	ɛ̃ə wʌʔ i ʔiː nĩ ŋna
	My mom throw uh. uh. Julie playdough out-away	māɪ mã oʊ wʌ̃ ʌ dʒuwi bēɪo õʊntʰ əweɪ		He eating a tug	ʔiʔiʔiː ə bʌŋ̊

FIGURE 1. A continuous speech sample from a child with delayed phonological development.

Historical and Theoretical Issues in Child Phonology

The Term Phonology

The term *phonology* is central in the shift from "articulation" to "phonological" disorders that has occurred in the last decade. Not all researchers have embraced this term or this shift. For example, in their excellent review paper, Shelton and McReynolds (1979) prefer to retain the term "articulation disorders." What really is meant when one refers to a child as having a phonological disorder in contrast to an articulation disorder?

Figure 2 is a conception that might be useful to contrast terminological differences and, perhaps, in so doing, to argue that the term "phonological disorders" is the more useful cover term for our interests. Figure 2 is a double-headed conception that portrays both the acquisition of speech— which normally takes place as a process between caregiver and child—and the intervention process when speech is delayed, which takes place between clinician and child. Management aspects of this figure will be discussed later. Essentially, we assume that what transpires between clinician and child should mirror what ordinarily transpires between caregiver and child. Here let us focus on the three tiers or boxes for the normal child as a language learner.

In the simplified conception in Figure 2, the business of phonology presumably transpires on at least three levels: a level of underlying representations of morphemes or words, a level for learning rules to combine morphemes and adjust features of sounds, and a level of manifest speech. What transpires at each of the levels is precisely the subject of linguistic inquiry, for only the surface level of manifest speech can be described directly. Speech pathologists are familiar with the descriptive devices at this lower or manifest level of speech. Analyses of manifest speech are covered in basic courses such as articulatory phonetics, acoustic phonetics, and all speech disorders courses. Moreover, when we use a standardized articulation test, we generally summarize manifest speech. That is, we tally and describe the errors a child exhibits relative to the ambient language.

When we venture into the upper two tiers in Figure 2, however, we require linguistic procedures for inferring mechanisms, basic units, and interrelations among speech forms and other aspects of the grammar. It is clear that some such level must be posited for the storage of speech and for certain combinatory processes that make speech production feasible and efficient. The confusion begins at these levels because linguistic journals are filled with dialogue about speech representation and generation. In fact, most conceptions of the child's developing system include many more levels of processing than the two basic levels portrayed in Figure 2 (see, for example, Smith, 1978; Macken, 1979). What is important to underscore here

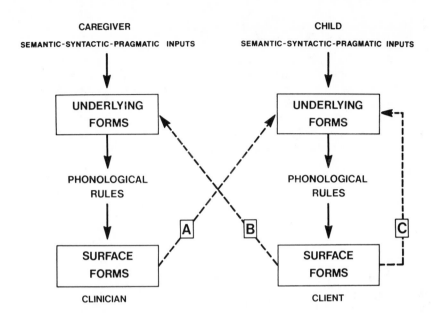

FIGURE 2. Elements in normal speech acquisition and intervention points for management.

is that some comprehensive view of the language user is what we mean by *phonology* in contrast to the term *articulation*. Those who concentrate solely on the articulatory and acoustic properties of their clients' speech sounds may be content to view the problem as one involving only peripheral aspects of the speech mechanism. In contrast, to the extent that assumptions are made about the child's organization of speech sounds—about how underlying forms for sounds and words and phonological errors are related to other components of the grammar—the clinician is thinking in the realm of phonology. Such clinicians may appropriately use the term *phonological disorders* in reference to their clients. A grossly overused metaphor, but one which is appropriate here, is that articulation is only the tip of the iceberg. And, for the task of working with young children with severely delayed speech, description of only this tip may be, at best, inefficient and, at worst, ineffective.

To summarize, the shift in terms from "articulation" to "phonology" reflects a more robust conception of the nature of speech delay. To many professionals, this shift is viewed as warranted because the speech errors seen at the manifest level are viewed as output from a system that must be understood before intervention issues can be addressed. For clients whose surface forms are not age-appropriate, the inquiry should be addressed to historical and concurrent workings of speech processing within a complex network represented in the upper tiers of Figure 2.

Phonological Theories

Figure 3 is a suggestive list that reminds us of the parent literature to which I have just alluded. Phonologists pursue issues related to the upper two tiers in Figure 2, as it is important to understand how sounds structure and function in natural languages of the world. Figure 3 includes a selected list of theorists who have proposed views that are the subject of lively debate in linguistic journals. Included in this list are some theories of phonology that must be considered basic sources for understanding normal and delayed acquisition of speech. Some of these theoretical positions are described in Dinnsen (1979). Persons who have not been following this literature should be mindful of its vitality. As in other areas of linguistics, small and large domain theories continually appear to challenge existing thought.

```
              THEORISTS:

         THE ORGANIZATION OF PHONOLOGY


    STRUCTURALISTS                  -- PRE-1950's
       (TAXONOMIC PHONEMICS)


    GENERATIVE PHONOLOGY            -- 1960's


    NATURAL GENERATIVE PHONOLOGY    -- LATE 1960's


    NATURAL PHONOLOGY               -- EARLY 1970's

    OTHERS:

       ATOMIC PHONOLOGY

       AUTOSEGMENTAL PHONOLOGY

       UPSIDE-DOWN PHONOLOGY
```

FIGURE 3. Approaches to phonology.

Figure 4 is a selective list of theorists, each of whom emphasizes different basic units in the study of normal child phonology. The point of this table is to remind us also of the flow of theoretical literature from which we derive our clinical concepts. At least one dozen major views on the processes and mechanisms of the acquisition of phonology are currently available (Ferguson and Garnica, 1975; Ferguson and Macken, 1980; Edwards and Shriberg, in preparation). These views differ from each other in major ways, in terms of their implications for theories of delayed phonological acquisition. The point here is only to remind us that the various approaches currently discussed in the literature on child phonology will continue to have an important influence on developing accounts of delayed phonological acquisition.

THEORISTS:
THE ACQUISITION OF PHONOLOGY

_____	--	PHONEME
JAKOBSON	--	FEATURE
BRANIGAN	--	SYLLABLE
STAMPE	--	NATURAL PROCESS
VIHMAN	--	PROSODY
WATERSON	--	SCHEMA
FERGUSON	--	WORD

FIGURE 4. Some theorists and basic units in the acquisition of phonology.

Phonological Analysis

A major focus in this volume is on alternative procedures for phonological analysis. Following is my approach to phonological analysis for children with developmental phonological disorders.

Five Types of Sound Change

Figure 5 contains a decision logic for describing speech behavior. Recall Dan's speech as shown in the clinician transcription sheet (Figure 1). A word-by-word inspection of Dan's speech would indicate that each word was either fully correct or that at least one sound in the word was different from the typical production expected from a child of his age. Let us call every example of the latter one type of *sound change*. Sound change can be defined as the difference between an underlying form (see Figure 2) and its realization as a surface form, i.e., manifest speech. The underlying form, in turn, is taken to be the broad phonemic transcription of a lexical item as given in a dictionary or, more appropriately, in a book such as Kenyon and Knott's *A Pronouncing Dictionary of American English* (1953). Let us divide sound changes into five categories as follows.

Type 1	Type 2	Type 3
Context-Sensitive Modifications	Context-Free Modifications	Phoneme Deletions and Substitutions
(a) Allophones (b) Casual and Fast Speech Changes	All place/manner changes that do not qualify as Type 1 modifications	(a) Natural Processes (b) Uncoded Deletions and Substitutions

FIGURE 5. Five types of sound change that occur in a continuous speech sample.

Context-Sensitive Modifications: Allophones—Type 1A. The first of the five types of sound change in Figure 5 (Type 1A) are commonly referred to as *allophones*. At the manifest speech level (see Figure 1) a /t/ is not a /t/ is not a /t/. Rather, low-level phonetic rules operating "downstream" of underlying forms convert (i.e. modify) abstract phonemes according to *context-sensitive* specifications. The phonetic description given in Kenyon and

Knott's phonetic dictionary is at a broad level. The phoneme /t/, for example, has a great many allophones or context-sensitive manifest forms that speakers normally use, including the alveolar flap [ɾ], e.g., *water* [wɑɾ ɚ]. Research by Zawadzki and Kuehn (1980), and others, suggests that there are at least two /r/ allophones that occur reliably in specific syllabic contexts. The problem is that some allophones are likely to be heard as an "error" by a clinician. For example, a velarized /l/ [ɫ] normally occurs post-vocalically, e.g., *tail* [tēɫ].[1] This allophone has not generally been discussed in phonetics books; hence, clinicians are likely to hear such context-sensitive modifications as incorrect. A child who says [tēɫ] should not, of course, be penalized for using a normally occurring adult allophone. On the contrary, use of proper allophones indicates emerging knowledge of not only under-lying forms, but also of the particular feature change rules that mark the dialect of the ambient language. As illustrated in Figure 2, only the activities of the middle box are presumably operative when a child changes an underlying phoneme to an appropriate output allophone. This is what is meant by the term *context-sensitive modification*.

Context-Sensitive Modifications: Casual and Fast Speech Changes— Type 1B.

The second type of context-sensitive modifications are sound changes that occur as acceptable forms in casual or fast speech. Unstressed words in casual or fast speech such as "bat and ball" [bæt n̩ bɑl], "ask her out" [æsk ɚ āῡt], are acceptable when reduced in this way. That is, such changes are sensitive to speech registers. When we take a free speech sample, we are hoping to obtain just this sort of "natural" speech. As with Type 1A changes, these sound changes also would be incorrectly consid-ered "wrong" in a phonological analysis. On the contrary, adjusting one's speech to a particular social level is pragmatically appropriate. Such sound changes are entirely fitting when one is speaking casually, provided that intelligibility is not compromised. Recognition of Type 1B sound changes is sometimes difficult. Elsewhere (Shriberg and Kwiatkowski, 1980), we present guidelines that allow us readily to type-sort such changes.

Context-Free Modifications: Type II.

The third type of sound change, *context-free modifications,* occurs in all phonetic contexts and in all speech

---

[1] Transcription symbolization follows Shriberg and Kent (1982). In this system, diphthongs are marked by an overbar, e.g., *eye* [āῑ].

registers. Hence, such changes are context-free. Among the distortions subsumed under Type II sound changes are: *dentalization* [ˏ], *derhotacization* [ᴜ] and *lateralization* [ᴖ]. Such sound changes, in my judgment, are conceptually distinct from the deletions and substitutions that characterize the remaining two types of sound change discussed below. Context-free modifications involve lower-level phonetic feature errors, rather than errors in the selection and inclusion of the correct underlying form. Conceptually, they are errors of feature specification at the same level as allophones. Whereas the modifications that occur in both Type I categories occur in selective places (i.e., context-sensitive), however, Type II sound changes occur in any context (context-free). Furthermore, the features used are generally not appropriate to any allophone of the phoneme. Lateralized /s/ [ʂ], for example, is not an allophone of /s/, nor is derhotacized /r/ [ɻ]. Whether or not such errors are handicapping to an individual is, of course, an entirely separate issue. Some children develop such context-free distortions and may retain them into adulthood. For assessment purposes, our task is to keep such sound change phenomena distinct from presumably higher-level linguistic processing "errors."

Deletions and Substitutions: Natural Phonological Processes— Type IIIA.

The fourth type of sound change introduces the somewhat infamous term, *natural phonological process.* Although a fully developed discussion of this construct is not appropriate here, it is important to take a brief look at some definitional issues. Following is a consolidated view of how our research group uses this construct for clinical purposes.

The concept of a natural phonological process is associated in the contemporary literature with the writings of David Stampe (1969, 1973; Donegan and Stampe, 1979). A natural phonological process is assumed to be an innate constraint on what is normally produced as manifest speech. As defined by Stampe, a natural phonological process works in the following way: given a potential phonological contrast, a process favors that member of the opposition which is least complex in terms of production, perception, or both. For example, given the choice of saying /w/ or /r/, the assumption is that /w/ is "easier." From this perspective, the simplification of /r/ that naturally occurs in children involves cognitive, perceptual, and production domains. For speech acquisition, the assumption is that children must learn to suppress such simplification in order to develop full productive control of the phonemes of the ambient language. A useful analogy might be to social behavior, wherein children must learn to suppress "what comes naturally."

That is, they must produce the appropriate social behavior for a particular context. What is central to this position is the notion that children already have an underlying representation of the appropriate target behavior. In Stampian terms, the natural process is a cover term for the phonological act of simplification. Hence, the child who deletes a final consonant in a word is thought to have "used" the natural phonological process of final consonant deletion. At such time as any final consonant is included, the child has "suppressed" use of this process. Again, the assumption is that the child does have an essentially adult-like underlying representation of the final consonant, and that the problem is one of increasing the constraints on the output phonology. Natural processes "explain" a child's final consonant deletions; cognitive constraints related to the pragmatics of communication presumably explain the dissolution of final consonant deletions (Campbell and Shriberg, in press).

There is continuing debate among phonologists, child phonologists, and those interested in clinical applications of Stampian notions about the use of such concepts. Dinnsen, Elbert, and Weismer (1979) have proposed guidelines to assess whether children have underlying representations of incorrect target behavior. McReynolds and Elbert (1981) have proposed qualitative and quantitative criteria for assessing when one might have sufficient evidence for the operation of phonological processes. Our theoretical and methodological position is discussed in detail elsewhere (Shriberg and Kwiatkowski, 1980). It is sufficient for the purposes of our discussion to note that the particular view of natural phonological processes we find most useful for clinical application is as follows.

We have identified eight putatively "natural" sound changes that meet the following specifications: (1) they involve phoneme deletions and/or substitutions rather than lower-level distortions, (2) they have face validity as sound changes that simplify speech production, (3) they are found frequently in children with delayed speech, and (4) they can be transcribed reliably by clinicians. The eight sound changes that meet these criteria are considered Type IIIA, natural phonological processes.

Deletions and Substitutions: Uncoded Processes—Type IIIB.   The fifth and final type of sound change, Type IIIB, is termed, simply, *Uncoded.* All other types of speech sound changes involving phoneme deletions and substitutions are viewed as speech sound change Type IIIB. For example, substitution of z/k, s/t, and r/d would appear odd, relative to any naturalness condition. Such sound changes do not happen in perceptual discrimination studies, nor do they occur when sound change is observed in a language over a period of time, nor do they generally occur in children developing speech normally, or in those with speech delays. Simply, these are the sound changes that do not meet the definitions for any of the other four types. By isolating them from the other four types of sound change, we set the stage for phonological analysis and for differential diagnosis. To illustrate such notions, let us now return to our opening case study and describe why we think Dan has such severely delayed phonological development.

Phonological Correlates of Middle-Ear Involvement

For a number of reasons, we suspected that Dan's speech was similar to the speech of a certain subgroup of children we have seen clinically—children with a history of middle-ear involvement. Dan's transcripts, as shown in Figure 1, indicated that he was making two types of Type IIIB sound changes, i.e., uncoded substitutions or deletions, which we also had begun to notice in children with histories of frequent middle-ear disease. These data (Shriberg and Smith, 1980) can briefly be summarized as follows.

Figure 6 describes two types of Type IIIB sound changes. The first sound change is actually a consolidation of three types of sound changes, wherein initial consonants are either deleted, replaced by [h], or replaced by [ʔ]. Examples for each type of sound change are listed in Figure 6. None of these sound changes are considered natural by our criteria. That is, by definition, they fall outside of our eight natural processes. Provisionally, then, they are sound changes that remain to be explained (Type IIIB).

The second type of sound change listed in Figure 6 is also a consolidated sound change, wherein nasal consonants are either substituted for

SOUND CHANGE	DESCRIPTION	EXAMPLES GLOSS	TRANSCRIPTION
I INITIAL CONSONANT CHANGE	INITIAL CONSONANTS ARE: –DELETED –REPLACED BY [h] –REPLACED BY [ʔ]	"GOT" "TIE" "TO"	[at] [haɪ] [ʔu]
II NASAL CONSONANT CHANGE	NASAL CONSONANTS ARE: –SUBSTITUTED FOR ONE ANOTHER –PARTIALLY DENASALIZED –REPLACED BY A STOP –PRECEDED/FOLLOWED BY AN EPENTHETIC STOP	"NOT" "KNEE" "MY" "NO"	[ma] [n̄iː] [ba] [dnðʊ]

FIGURE 6. Two Type IIIB sound change classes (see Figure 5).

one another, partially denasalized, replaced by a stop, or preceded or followed by an epenthetic stop. Again, notice the examples for each in Figure 6. We assume that such changes fall into our default class. That is, they cannot be sorted into one of the other four sound changes, so they are labeled Type IIIB, Uncoded.

What we observed in children with middle-ear involvement histories is that one or both of these sound change categories occur frequently in their transcripts. We set about to do a controlled study of the prevalence of such changes in the speech of children with delayed phonological acquisition who had histories of middle-ear involvement in contrast to children with delayed speech who were not so involved. Figure 7 presents the descriptive statistics for two groups that we assembled for this purpose. The two groups of 11 children were similar in age, severity of involvement, and mean length of utterance. Figure 8 illustrates the results of our inspection of the occasion of Sound Change I and Sound Change II in the speech of both groups of speech-delayed children. It is apparent visually and was readily confirmed statistically that Sound Change I and II occurred more frequently in children who had positive histories for middle-ear involvement. We have cross-vali-

VARIABLE	MIDDLE-EAR INVOLVEMENT			NON MIDDLE-EAR INVOLVEMENT		
	$\bar{x}$	SD	RANGE	$\bar{x}$	SD	RANGE
AGE	54.7	10.3	42-72	63.9	7.3	49-74
SEVERITY**	61.7	13.3	43-81	63.6	7.8	52-74
MLU	3.2	1.1	1.5-5.2	3.5	1.4	1.5-6.9

*N=11 FOR EACH GROUP, WITH 9 AND 8 MALES IN THE MIDDLE-EAR INVOLVEMENT GROUP AND THE NON-MIDDLE-EAR INVOLVEMENT GROUP, RESPECTIVELY.

**SEVERITY VALUES ARE THE PERCENTAGE OF CONSONANTS CORRECT IN THE CONTINUOUS SPEECH SAMPLE.

FIGURE 7. Descriptive statistics for two groups of speech-delayed children.

dated these data in another sample of speech delayed children provided by Dr. Barbara Hodson. These data presented in Figure 8 are important to pursue, for middle-ear disease may be a factor contributing to delayed speech (Shriberg, in press, b). In the present context, however, the focus is on methodology. The five-category sort of sound changes represent our interpretation of Stampian notions and an arbitrary definitional stance for the purposes of clinical application. This approach did allow us to sift from among the "errors" of children with delayed speech, certain sound changes for inspection. Let us now proceed to illustrate how such procedures form only one component in a system for provisional diagnostic classification of children with developmental phonological disorders.

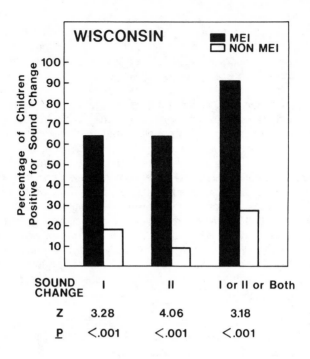

FIGURE 8. Percentage of children in each group scored positive for one or both sound changes.

Diagnostic Classification of Developmental Phonological Disorders

One challenge to any worker charged with the task of synthesis is to reduce a universe of inquiry to one 8½ by 11 sheet of paper. Our current version of a response to this challenge is shown as Figure 9. Figure 9 is a form for classifying children who have a developmental phonological disorder. At the highest level of the system, the child is classified as having, or not having, a phonological disorder. For children with a phonological disorder, successively lower levels of the worksheet provide increasingly more descriptive detail. This system, which is fully described elsewhere (Shriberg and Kwiatkowski, in press, a), provides a means by which researchers and clinicians can organize, store, and retrieve assessment data. Our research goals include an eventual genetic classification system (Shriberg, in press, a). The emphasis here is to illustrate in a general way how the system works,

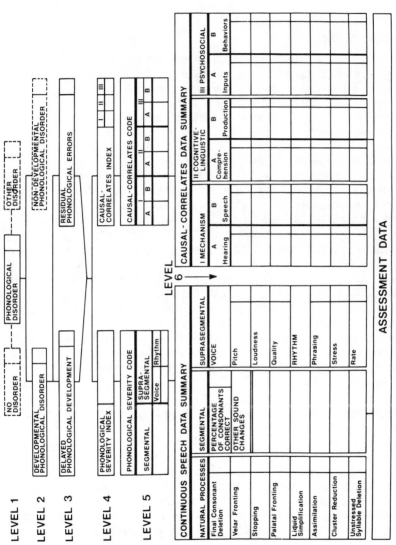

FIGURE 9. A summary form for diagnostic classification of children with a developmental phonological disorder.

including the role played by phonological process information. For convenience, we will work up the levels shown in Figure 9. Notice that the system branches into two summary components: the speech data and the causal correlates data.

Speech Data

Classification of a child or an adult begins with the assessment data (see Fig. 9, bottom box) that feed the system. Any person with a suspected speech problem is referred and assessed. Depending upon the presenting problems and the myriad of individual differences among clinicians and employment sites, a battery of assessment measures is constructed and administered. We favor use of a continuous speech sample from which three types of data may be derived for the speech branch at Level 6 of the classification worksheet.

The speech branch at Level 6 is divided into three sections: natural processes, segmental data, and suprasegmental data. The object is to describe and code data from the continuous speech sample in each of these three major subdivisions.

Natural Process Data. Natural process data are coded by means of a procedure designed expressly for continuous speech (Shriberg and Kwiatkowski, 1980). As before, we code eight sound-change categories that are well-attested to as natural, frequent in children with delayed speech, and capable of being reliably scored. Following instructions in the reference publication, a check is placed in the box beside each process (see Figure 9) if a process is evident at least some time in the continuous speech sample. Obviously this "check" is itself summary information. As with all information on this diagnostic classification form, the relevant details exist only at the level of the assessment data itself.

Segmental Data. The next subcategory, segmental data, provides space to record two types of information. A percentage of consonants correct score is derived from the continuous speech sample following a procedure described in Shriberg and Kwiatkowski (in press, c). Use of this percentage will be described shortly. The remaining boxes in the segmental data section are for recording all sound changes not coded as natural processes. With reference to Figure 5, these include all Type II sound changes (context-free distortions) and Type IIIB sound changes (deletions and substitutions not coded as one of the eight natural processes).

Suprasegmental Data. The third subcategory of data taken from the continuous speech sample codes a child's suprasegmental behaviors. Suprasegmental behaviors are divided into two main sections, Voice and

Rhythm. Voice includes pitch, loudness and quality. Rhythm includes phrasing, stress and rate. For each of these six suprasegmentals, a clinician judges whether the client is within the normal limits, or is deviant from normal "a few times" during the speech sample (less than 20% of utterances), or "often" during the speech sample (greater than 20% of utterances). A *0, 1, 2* ordinal system is used to specify these distinctions, wherein *0* = normal for the linguistic, pragmatic context, *1* = slight to pronounced deviation from normal occurring *a few times* during the sample, and *2* = slight to pronounced deviation from normal occurring *often* during the sample. As described in the reference publication, a percentage-of-occurrence base was more reliable than a magnitude-estimation base for the purpose of relating suprasegmentals to severity (to be discussed shortly).

Summary of Speech Branch. Notice that in these three sections—natural processes, segmental data, and suprasegmental data—we have gleaned from the continuous speech sample a wealth of descriptive and diagnostic information. In keeping with our opening remarks, we view these speech data as only one of two major pieces of assessment information. The other side of the picture, literally the right branch in Figure 9, provides for a worksheet summary of other types of information normally obtained in an assessment process.

Causal-Correlates Data

A second assessment concern is to explore all extra-linguistic factors that may be causally associated or correlated with past and present speech deficits. In Figure 9, the right-hand branch of the classification system provides a format for reducing and quantifying these assessment data. For the task of organizing, storing, and retrieving causal-correlates data, a conception of three major areas is proposed: Mechanism, Cognitive-Linguistic, and Psychosocial. These areas, in turn, are each subdivided into two categories as shown in Figure 9. Essentially, the clinician's task is to reduce information in each of these areas by means of a three-way coding decision: *1* = normal, unremarkable; *2* = questionable or mild involvement; *3* = moderate to severe involvement. This simple coding system is used to code all data from an assessment battery in the appropriate columns listed in the causal-correlates section in Figure 9.

Causal-Correlates I: Mechanism Factors. The first section in the causal-correlates branch of the worksheet is divided into two sub-areas, (A) Hearing and (B) Speech. Within each subdivision, respectively, the structural and functional adequacy of hearing and speech mechanisms is assessed by means of perceptual and instrumental measures. The particular perceptual and instrumental procedures used for these analyses depend on the training of the examiner and available facilities. For example, whereas acoustic immittance measures have become routine in most clinical settings, aerodynamic measures have not. The 1980s will undoubtedly see major emphasis placed upon simple, reliable instrumental approaches to the assessment of neuromuscular systems. Currently, however, the oral-peripheral examination provides the speech mechanism information, with case history data (e.g., developmental data, medical history) and audiological findings providing information that may contribute to the causal-correlates picture. Overall, the clinician-researcher is interested in documenting any historical and/or maintaining factors that may delimit speech perception or production.

Causal-Correlates II: Cognitive-Linguistic Factors. The second causal-correlates section in Figure 9 reflects the effect of a person's cognitive-linguistic function on phonological development. The subdivisions are (A) Comprehension and (B) Production. In this assessment, too, theoretical and methodological differences are widely debated (Miller, 1981); no single protocol has gained consensus. Whichever the particular assessment measures used, a certain proportion of children with phonological disorders have cognitive-linguistic deficits that are important causal or contributing factors.

Causal-Correlates III: Psychosocial Factors. Psychosocial functioning is perhaps the least well-described area in diagnostic classification. Subcategory A, Input, includes information on caregivers, home, school, and other sources of input to the child's psychosocial development. Subcategory B, Behaviors, allows for rating of the child's overt performance in these different settings.

Summary Levels

Once data are coded at Level 6 for the speech and the causal-correlates data, completing all remaining levels of the system is essentially a clerical task. Level 5 causal-correlates entries are simply the highest number for any individual entry at Level 6. Similarly, suprasegmental entries at Level 5 reflect the highest recorded entry for voice and rhythm at Level 6. The larger box for segmental information is completed with reference to conversions listed in Shriberg and Kwiatkowski (in press, c). In that study, we present validation data for a four-term adjective system for specifying severity of involvement. The percentage of correct consonants as given at Level 6 in the segmental data is converted into one of the four adjectives, *mild, mild-moderate, moderate-severe,* or *severe.* The information coded at Level 4, again, simply reduces further the information at Level 5. For the causal-correlates index, the highest number in each of the boxes at Level 5 is carried upwards. For the speech branch, a severity adjective is entered in the box for a phonological severity index according to directions given in the reference publication. Finally, Levels 2 and 3 of the diagnostic classification sheet provide for a distinction between developmental phonological disorders and non-developmental phonological disorders (Level 2) and delayed phonological development versus residual phonological errors (Level 3). The distinction at Level 3 is basically one of age and the type of phonological pattern. Young children who have natural process errors are considered to have *delayed phonological development.* Older children with distortion errors are classified as having *residual phonological errors.* These matters are detailed in Shriberg and Kwiatkowski (in press, a). A developmental phonological disorder, as indicated at Level 2, is distinguished from non-developmental phonological disorders on the basis of the age of onset. There are those individuals who report to the clinic having had speech errors concomitant with accidents, and other causes, occurring past the developmental period. While such errors eventually may be topographically similar to those seen in children with developmental phonological disorders, the fact that they occur after the developmental period has important implications for management strategies.

Sample Completed Classification Form.   Figure 10 is an example of a completed diagnostic classification form. In practice, somewhat more detail is preserved at Level 6 than can be illustrated here. To review this information, notice that this child is classified as having a developmental phonological disorder (Level 2), delayed phonological development (Level 3), severe involvement (Level 4), with a causal-correlates code of 221 (Level 4). The speech data indicate that her speech contains instances of six of eight natural processes as well as many Type II sound changes (context-free modifications) and Type IIIB changes (uncoded deletions and substitutions). She was also given ratings of 2 on the Voice suprasegmentals of pitch and quality. Her causal-correlates data summary indicates some non-0 entries in four of the six causal-correlates columns. Again, detailed assessment information is contained in the assessment materials that are used to generate the abbreviated entries in Figure 10. A table in Shriberg and Kwiatkowski (in press, a) provides approximately 100 descriptors that were used in a study (described next) of the diagnostic classification system. As shown in Figure 10, this young girl had 1 and 2 ratings in a number of these assessment categories.

Some Preliminary Data

A study of the diagnostic classification system has been accomplished on a retrospective sample of 43 children with delayed speech. These data (Shriberg and Kwiatkowski, in press, a) are summarized in Figure 11. Briefly, within Mechanism variables, we see that only one-third of the children had a clearly unremarkable hearing or speech mechanism history, or status. Two-thirds of the children earned codes of 1 or 2, indicating either questionable or demonstrable involvement in these areas. For Cognitive-Linguistic vari-

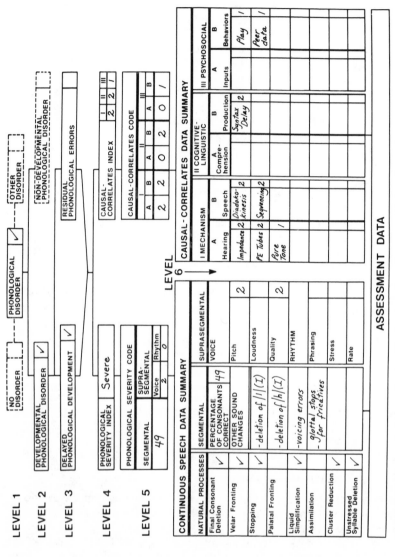

FIGURE 10. A sample diagnostic classification form for a five-year-old girl referred for assessment of her "intelligibility" problems.

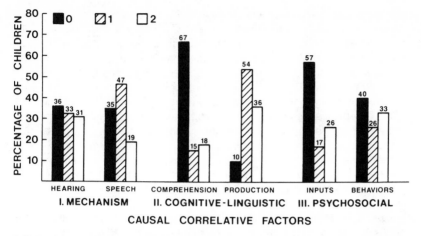

FIGURE 11. Causal-correlates data for a group of 43 children with delayed speech.

ables, comprehension was rated as normal for two-thirds of the children; not unexpectedly, only 10 percent of the children were seen as normal in productive language. Finally, our psychosocial data suggest that from 40 to 60 percent of the children have questionable to severe histories or current involvement in either inputs or behaviors. We view these data as preliminary. They have guided our research program, as demonstrated in the case example of Dan. Eventually, we will be interested in matching children's diagnostic assessment coding to management programs, a topic we turn to now for brief comment.

Intervention Points for Management

It seems clear from the current literature in phonological disorders that no one management approach has proven superiority over others (Shelton and McReynolds, 1979). Our own efforts to deal with both the form and the content of management (Shriberg and Kwiatkowski, in press, b) indicate strongly that a "universal" management program is probably an unrealistic goal. Rather, we suspect that effective and efficient programs will need to be tailored to the child in very specific ways. Let us look at one parameter within which current and future intervention programs differ sharply, a parameter we term entry points for intervention.

Entry Points for Intervention

Figure 2, as you recall, is a representation of the basic components of the acquisition of phonology and of the management process. The assumption is that management, in general, mirrors normal acquisition. Attention is here drawn to the small boxes labeled A, B, and C in Figure 2. Each box indicates a possible intervention point for children with delayed phonological acquisition. We currently view distinctions among these points as central to a theory-into-practice approach to management programming.

As positioned in this representation of normal speech acquisition (Figure 2), the child's initial task is to establish underlying forms for the surface forms of the caregiver's language. The learning task eventuates in comprehension of English phonology. Comprehension of English phonology requires adequate functioning of process constructs such as *attention, perception, identification, recognition,* and *discrimination.* One way to teach phonology to a child who has not naturally acquired it is to focus intervention at just this point, represented as Entry Point A. Therapy procedures requiring the child to attend, listen, discriminate, monitor, and so forth, are at the core of traditional speech therapy. In fact, from the "ear-training" approaches of the 1930s to the "auditory processing" programs of the 1970s, Entry Point A intervention programs have enjoyed favor by generations of clinicians.

A second point of intervention for children with phonological delay is at Entry Point B, in Figure 2. The child's task here is to *produce* speech behavior, which then is judged for its correctness by a clinician or, perhaps, nowadays, by some signal-recognition device. Intervention at this point focuses on speech production, in contrast to the speech comprehension focus of Entry Point A. Speech production focus was popular in the very earliest, "drill" period of speech therapy and became prominent again in the behavioral emphasis of the 1960s.

The point of intervention represented as Entry Point C, in Figure 2, requires both that the child produce speech and make some sort of comprehension response. Translated to a typical clinical activity, a child might be rewarded differently if he or she produces a speech target correctly and also discerns whether or not the sound was made correctly.

Issues in Intervention

What implications do these alternative entry points have for issues in management programming? Three interrelated issues may be addressed: necessary/sufficient issues, sequencing issues, and target selection issues.

Necessary/Sufficient Issues. The necessary/sufficient issues reflect the choice clinicians have in selecting from among programs that emphasize one or more points of intervention. Programs that stress comprehension activities located at Entry Point A (e.g., Winitz, 1975), the production activities at Entry Point B (e.g., McCabe and Bradley, 1975), or the production-comprehension activities at Entry Point C (e.g., Weiner and Ostrowski, 1979), have all reported successful acquisition data. We have few data, however, on whether management at any one of these points alone is a *sufficient* therapy. The point here is that normal phonological development evidently progresses to some form of Point C processing, without the child experiencing explicit contingencies at Point A or Point B. Is management focused at Point A or Point B necessary for children with delayed phonological acquisition? Is management at Point C sufficient for children with delayed phonological acquisition? Finding the answers to such questions will require a comprehensive research effort.

Sequencing Issues.   A second, and interrelated, issue concerns the sequence of entry points. If programming of all three types needs to be provided, should the progression A-B-C always be programmed in sequence? Specifically, should we always have children engage in management activities that follow the sequence: (1) comprehension of others; (2) self-production; and (3) self-production and comprehension of self? Inspection of published management programs indicates that just such a sequence is typical of published programs dating back to the 1930s (Shriberg and Kwiatkowski, in press, *b*). Aside from the efficiency issue addressed above, one could argue for intervention that began with Entry Point C activities, only later to progress to Point B. For example, consider a management program for a child who is deleting final consonants. If we begin management asking a child to key in on whether or not he or she deleted consonants in a target stimulus, we immediately press the child to "tune in." Weiner and Ostrowski (1979) describe just such a procedure. The procedure requires that the child accomplish very taxing perceptual-cognitive operations in the comprehension domain, particularly in memory. For certain children, perhaps those more involved in comprehension domains (i.e., Figure 9, Type IIA), such activities may actualize necessary processes. Note that the alternative points require far less linguistic processing. In an over-simplified sense, Entry Point A activities do not involve the child's output phonology (unless one adheres to a motor theory of speech perception), while Entry Point B activities do not involve a child's perceptual phonology. Entry Point C approaches presumably involve both. Again, such issues are closely tied to theories of normal and delayed phonological acquisition. If at least some delayed-speech children have difficulty organizing input-output phonologies, the intervention sequence might better start at Entry Point C. Activity at Point A and Point B would then be reserved for later teaching of new target behaviors. Certainly, when the focus switches to phonetic events, such as fine-tuning a child's residual articulation errors, response development at Point A and Point B is warranted.

Target Selection Issues.   As suggested in the last sentence above, a third and interrelated issue in programming concerns target selection. Whichever the target—whether selected from among units the size of a feature, a sound, or a sound-change process—we have the choice of teaching at Points A, B, or C. Target selection issues are extremely complex, currently, for we have so many theories of acquisition from which to formulate a rationale. During the long era of structuralist theory, we routinely taught sounds; we then switched to features; lately we have been trying phonological processes. How might unit selection, and selection of a particular target within that unit, interact with choice of an intervention point?

With reference to natural processes as a target unit, I would submit that Point C intervention is the only one of the three that is appropriate. The concept of process "suppression," introduced earlier, is fundamental here. If the assumption is that a child really is capable of correct output, but is not actively suppressing the disposition to simplify, then Point C provides the appropriate intervention experience. Point A intervention assumes that underlying forms need to be established or perhaps better defined—which is not the case, as argued by Stampe. Point B intervention assumes that surface forms need to be modified in topography, which is not the relevant issue for children with delayed speech. Only Point C assumes that the child has the capacity to produce the correct form, but that cognitive processes are not sufficiently engaged to motivate correct speech production. Notice that if one assumes that perception or production of a sound or feature *itself* is being taught, then intervention at Point A and Point B is an appropriate arrangement of teaching events. If what is being taught is increasing disposition to suppress the tendency to simplify complex articulatory targets, however, then only Point C programs address the relevant cognitive mechanisms.

Conclusions

I have tried to present two bodies of information. Overall, I have tried to integrate some terms in phonology with particular emphasis on the relationship of theory to assessment. Also, I have introduced a diagnostic classification system that integrates linguistic and extra-linguistic data. Eventual development of the system is predicated on the assumption that sub-groups of children with developmental phonological disorders may be identified. I have presented preliminary data on one such group—children with a history of middle-ear involvement. Implications of these classification categories for differential management programming remain a challenging long-term research goal.

References

Bankson, N. Whatever happened to functional articulation disorders? Paper presented to the Annual Convention of the American Speech-Language-Hearing Association, Detroit, November 1980.

Campbell, T., and Shriberg, L. Associations among pragmatic functions, lexical stress, and phonological processes in children with delayed phonological development. *Journal of Speech and Hearing Research,* (In press).

Dinnsen, D. *Current Approaches to Phonological Theory.* Bloomington, Indiana: Indiana University Linguistics Club, 1979.

Dinnsen, D., Elbert, M., and Weismer, G. On the characterization of functional misarticulation. Paper presented to the Annual Convention of the American Speech-Language-Hearing Association, Atlanta, 1979.

Donegan, P., and Stampe, D. The study of natural phonology. In D. Dinnsen (Ed.) *Current Approaches to Phonological Theory,* Bloomington, Indiana: Indiana University Linguistics Club, 1979.

Edwards, M., and Shriberg, L. *Phonological Theory: History and Applications in Communication Disorders.* In preparation.

Ferguson, C. and Garnica, O. Theories of phonological development. In E. Lenneberg and E. Lenneberg (Eds.) *Foundations of Language Development* II, New York: Academic Press, 1975.

Ferguson, C. and Macken, M. Phonological development in children: play and cognition. *Papers and Reports on Child Language Development,* 1980, *18,* 138–177.

Kenyon, J. and Knott, T. *A Pronouncing Dictionary of American English.* Springfield, Massachusetts: Merriam, 1953.

McCabe, R. and Bradley D. Systematic multiple phonemic approach to articulation therapy. *Acta Symolica,* 1975, *6,* 1–18.

Miller, J. (Ed.) *Assessing Language Production in Children: Experimental Procedures.* Baltimore: University Park Press, 1981.

Macken, M. The child's lexical representation: The 'puzzle-puddle-pickle' evidence. *Papers and Reports on Child Language Development,* 1979, *16,* 26–41.

McReynolds, L. and Elbert, M. Criteria for phonological analysis. *Journal of Speech and Hearing Disorders,* 1981, *46,* 197–204.

Shelton, R., and McReynolds, L. Functional articulation disorders: preliminaries to treatment. In N. Lass (Ed.) *Speech and Language: Advances in Basic Research and Practice, 2,* New York: Academic Press, Inc., 1979.

Shriberg, L. A response evocation program for / ɝ /. *Journal of Speech and Hearing Disorders,* 1975, *40,* 92–105.

Shriberg, L. An intervention procedure for children with persistent /r/ errors. *Language Speech and Hearing Services in Schools,* 1980, *11,* 102–110.

Shriberg, L. Towards classification of developmental phonological disorders. In N. Lass (Ed.) *Speech and Language: Advances in Basic Research and Practice,* VIII, New York: Academic Press Inc. (In press, *a*).

Shriberg, L. Correlates of recurrent otitis media in children with developmental phonological disorders. In R. Naremore (Ed.) *Implications of Otitis Media for Speech and Language Development.* New York: Brian C. Decker (In press, *b*).

Shriberg, L. and Kent, R. *Clinical Phonetics.* New York: John Wiley and Sons, 1982.

Shriberg, L. and Kwiatkowski, J. *Natural Process Analysis (NPA): A Procedure for Phonological Analysis of Continuous Speech Samples.* New York: John Wiley and Sons, 1980.

Shriberg, L. and Kwiatkowski, J. Phonological disorders I: A diagnostic classification system. *Journal of Speech and Hearing Disorders* (In press, *a*).

Shriberg, L. and Kwiatkowski, J. Phonological disorders II: A conceptual framework for management. *Journal of Speech and Hearing Disorders* (In press, *b*).

Shriberg, L. and Kwiatkowski, J. Phonological disorders III: A metric for assessing severity of involvement. *Journal of Speech and Hearing Disorders* (In press, *c*).

Shriberg, L. and Smith, A. Phonological correlates of middle-ear involvement in children with delayed speech. Paper presented to the Annual Convention of the American Speech-Language-Hearing Association, Detroit, 1980.

Smith, N. Lexical representation and the acquisition of phonology. Forum lecture at the Linguistic Society of American Institute, Urbana, Illinois, 1978.

Stampe, D. The acquisition of phonetic representation. Papers from the Fifth Regional Meeting, Chicago Linguistic Society, 1969.

Stampe, D. A dissertation on natural phonology. Unpublished doctoral dissertation, University of Chicago, 1973.

Weiner, F. and Ostrowski, A. Effects of listener uncertainty on articulation inconsistency. *Journal of Speech and Hearing Disorders,* 1979, *44,* 487–493.

Winitz, H. *From Syllable to Conversation.* Baltimore: University Park Press, 1975.

Zawadzki, P. and Kuehn, D. A cineradiographic study of static and dynamic aspects of American English /r/. *Phonetics,* 1980, *37,* 253–266.

4 Minimal Word-Pairs and Distinctive Feature Training

Stephen E. Blache

Purpose of Presentation

In this presentation, I hope to develop a detailed orientation to the clinical utilization of distinctive features (sound substitution or sound class processes—as they are called today). My ultimate goal is to establish a foundation that is comprehensive enough to enable a therapist to use distinctive features in everyday clinical settings.

Method of Presentation

To accomplish my goal, the presentation will be broken down into four sections. The first section will concentrate on what distinctive features are. This will be followed by a discussion of how distinctive features may be used in training. The third section will be devoted to the organization of the distinctive features and the procedures used in the selection of the training goals for the individual child. The presentation will conclude with a discussion of the background testing that should accompany each training program. In all, we will learn how to make features distinctive. We will learn in what order features should be selected for training. Finally, we will learn how to determine when a distinctive feature orientation is the best approach to therapy.

The Distinctive Feature

A distinctive feature is any sound property that makes words different.[1] To illustrate this phenomenon, I offer the following example (see Figure 1): here, we have two words represented—"T" and "key." The words are separated by a single distinctive feature, commonly referred to as front/back tongue placement, compact/diffuse, or some other such term.

---

[1] A phoneme is defined as "a *set* of concurrent sound properties which are used in a given language to *distinguish words of unlike meaning* (Jakobson, 1962, p. 261; cf. Blache, 1978a; Compton, 1970; Singh, 1976; Walsh, 1974; Winitz, 1969)." By implication, any member of the set, i.e. feature, may distinguish words, i.e. be distinctive.

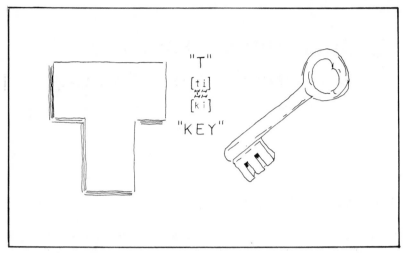

FIGURE 1. An exemplar illustrating the representation of a front/back lingual contrast occurring in the initial segmental position. (The phonetic code typically is omitted from the card.)

Front versus Back Tongue Placement

If a child can hear the difference between the pronunciation of "T" and "key," we assume that the child is sensitive to variations in closure of the oral cavity at the position of the tongue tip versus the back-tongue point of articulation. Conversely, if a child can actively control the closure of the oral cavity at the position of the tongue tip and the back-tongue position, the acoustic end-products will trigger a linguistic difference in the ear of the listener. In all, distinctive features are sets of consistent motoric gestures that result in acoustic end-products that can be recognized as being linguistically different by another listener. Every distinctive feature has a physiological component, an acoustical component, a psychological component, a cultural component, and a differential component.

Minimal Word-Pairs.   If we look at the phonetic transcription of our two words, we will notice that both words have an equal number of segments. Each of the two words has two sounds in it. The distinctive feature contrast occurs in the initial position—[t] is opposing [k]. The difference between the two sounds, [t] and [k], is 'minimal' because a single sound property separates the two sounds. When two words are essentially identical, and they differ by one feature or sound property, we say the words are 'minimal-pair' words.

Non-Minimal Word-Pairs.   Examining the 19 consonantal sounds of American English, it can be noted that more than one distinctive feature can separate two sounds (see Table 1). In the current approach, six distinctive

TABLE 1 The Number of Distinctive Feature Differences Separating the Consonants of American English

Target	REFERENCE SOUND																		
	p	f	b	v	m	t	θ	s	d	ð	z	n	k	tʃ	ʃ	g	dʒ	ʒ	ŋ
[p]	..p	1	1	2	2	1	2	3	2	3	4	3	2	3	4	3	4	5	4
[f]	......f		2	1	3	2	1	2	3	2	3	4	3	2	3	4	3	4	5
[b]	.........b			1	1	2	3	4	1	2	3	2	3	4	5	2	3	4	3
[v]	v				2	3	2	3	2	1	2	3	4	3	4	3	2	3	4
[m]	..................m					3	4	5	2	3	4	1	4	5	6	3	4	5	2
[t]	.......................t						1	2	1	2	3	2	1	2	3	2	3	4	3
[θ]	...........................θ							1	2	1	2	3	2	1	2	3	2	3	4
[s]	..............................s								3	2	1	4	3	2	1	4	3	2	5
[d]	..................................d									1	2	1	2	3	4	1	2	3	2
[ð]	......................................ð										1	2	3	2	3	2	1	2	3
[z]	....z											3	4	3	2	3	2	1	4
[n]	....n												3	4	5	2	3	4	1
[k]	....k													1	2	1	2	3	2
[tʃ]	....tʃ														1	2	1	2	3
[ʃ]	....ʃ															3	2	1	4
[g]	....g																1	2	1
[dʒ]	....dʒ																	1	2
[ʒ]	....ʒ																		3

(Blache, 1978, p. 252)

features are used to separate the consonants: nasality, voicing, front place, stridency, continuation and back place. On the first line of the table, it is noted that [p] is different from [t]. This difference is based on the front place (lip versus tongue) contrast. This is a minimal difference. When [p] is contrasted to [ʃ], 'sh,' at the end of the first line, there are four features separating the two sounds. The number of feature differences between consonants may vary from 1 to 6. In distinctive feature training, we will use only those sound pairs or couplets that are separated by a single distinctive feature. This is what is implied by the term 'minimal.'

Why use minimal-pairs? Part of our training task involves discrimination testing. If our two words are separated by two features, we will have a problem. As the therapist randomly pronounces the two words, the child is asked to indicate the proper picture. If the words involve two features, the child may respond correctly using either of the features. The therapist will not know whether one, or the other, or both, features are being used with the child's response. By using a single distinctive feature, this problem is avoided.

Referring to Table 1, it can be noted that there are 33 pure (single feature) contrasts among the 171 possible sound-pair couplets. Three of the 33 involve nasality, 8 of the 33 involve voicing, 5 of the 33 involve front place, 4 of the 33 involve stridency, 6 of the 33 involve continuation, and 7 of the 33 involve back place. In the course of this presentation, we will examine the organization of these 33 contrasts until they become quite familiar. These 33 contrasts or distinctive features are the goals of therapeutic training.

Front Place (Labial/Lingual) Contrast

Let us look at some representative minimal-pairs for each of the six features. We have looked at the front versus back tongue contrast with "T" and "key." In the next example, [p] is opposing [t] (see Figure 2b). This contrast emphasizes the importance of the use of the lips versus the use of the tongue tip. Sounds made by the lips have a low pitch; sounds made by the tongue tip have a much higher pitch. If you will say [p] and [t] to yourself, you will notice this difference. The motoric gesture produces the contrasting acoustic signals. These signals are used to differentiate words in specific cultures, by individuals at a psychological level.

In traditional approaches, we have taught children to make sounds. In a distinctive feature approach, the ultimate goal is to teach the child to differentiate between words, i.e., produce distinctiveness. The components of the speech sounds, the features, are the tools of differentiation. In this approach, we will always work at the word level. We will contrast sounds in such a way that the individual distinctive features are isolated.

Voiced/Voiceless Contrast

The minimal-pair words "pear"–"bear" isolate the voicing contrast (see Figure 2c). To use this feature, the child must be able to understand the importance of the presence or absence of laryngeal activity. It can be noted that these minimal-pair words have three sound segments. The contrast occurs in the initial position. The second and third segments, the vowel and the [r], are identical. Minimal-pair words may be of any length. The important thing is that all but one segment be identical.

Nasal/Non-Nasal Contrast

With the contrast "bunny"–"money," we have words with 4 segments (see Figure 2d). Three of the four segments are identical. The distinctive feature contrast occurs in the initial position, where [b] opposes [m]. Actually, the contrast may occur in any position in the word. For instance, "slab"–"slam" will serve as minimal-pair words for the [b–m] contrast in the final position. The presence or absence of nasality is still the key element that separates the two words.

The difference between [b] and [m] is triggered by an opening and closing of the velopharyngeal port. If the velum is left in a lowered position, nasal resonance is produced by the nasal cavity. If the velum is raised, nasal resonance is eliminated, and the [m] reverts to [b].

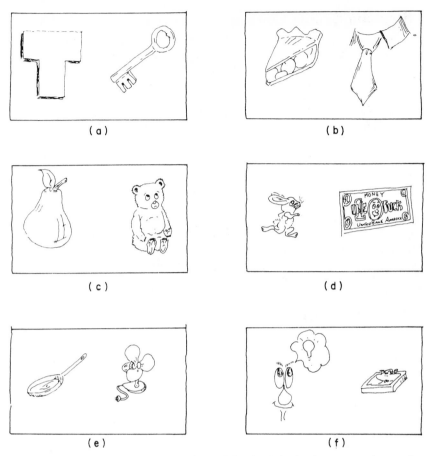

(a) (b)

(c) (d)

(e) (f)

FIGURE 2. Six exemplars illustrating each of the six distinctive features used to teach the consonants and/or semivowels. (Note that the contrasting words must be of equal segmental length, but they may vary in length from word-pair to word-pair.)

Continued/Interrupted Contrast

In our next example, [p] is opposing [f] (see Figure 2e). The difference between "pan" and "fan" is based on the fact that [p] is articulated briefly. The [f], on the other hand, is produced using a longer posture. This is the continued/interrupted feature. By tradition, each distinctive feature has an acoustic and a physiological definition (Blache, 1970). The time it takes to produce the signal, and the length of the acoustic end-product are significant linguistic cues in our culture.

Strident/Mellow Contrast

In our final example, "think"–"sink," the mellow characteristics of the voiceless 'th' $[\theta]$, are contrasted to the strident qualities of 's,' $[s]$ (see Figure 2f). Children who are not sensitive to this contrast may have an interdental lisp. This condition may be produced by poor understanding, poor motoric control, poor hearing abilities, a poor speech model in the home, poor motivation to develop linguistic skills, slow intellectual development, and/or structural inadequacy. These same causes of deficit may also affect the previous five features.

Summary

In all, to produce consonants, the child must understand place of articulation: the lips versus the tongue—the front of the tongue versus the back of the tongue. These two features produce three points of articulation; the lips, the tongue-tip, and the back of the tongue. The child must also understand manner of articulation characteristics. The spectral requirements of nasality and voicing must be integrated and the aerodynamic requirements of continuation and stridency must be fathomed and controlled.

The Phonemic Model

In Figure 3, you will see a model of the 6 features, and the manner in which they separate the 19 consonants. Nasality can be seen as the lines that separate $[b/m]$, $[d/n]$ and $[g/\eta]$. Voicing separates $[p/b]$, $[f/v]$, $[t/d]$, $[\theta/\eth]$, $[s/z]$, $[k/g]$, $[t\int/d\mathsf{z}]$ and $[\int/\mathsf{z}]$. Notice that all the sounds on the bottom of the figure are voiceless: $p, f, t, \theta, s, k, t\int,$ and $\int$. Immediately above each of these sounds are the voiced counterparts of the voiceless set. The ceiling of the first story (so to speak), or the floor of the second story, is made up of voiced sounds: $b, v, d, \eth, z, g, d\mathsf{z},$ and z. Finally, three voiced sounds $[b/d/g]$ have nasal counterparts, $[m/n/\eta]$. At the top of the model we have nasals, lower down are the voiced sounds, and on the bottom of the model we have the voiceless sounds. Two features, nasality and voicing, separate the three classes.

From left to right are the distinctive features that relate to place of articulation. At the far left wall, we have five labial sounds: $m, b, p, f,$ and v. All the remaining sounds, to the right, involve the use of the tongue. $[m/n]$, $[b/d]$, $[p/t]$, $[f/\theta]$, and $[v/\eth]$ are sound couplets that emphasize the labial/lingual or front place contrast. Seven sounds in the middle of the model use tongue-tip emphasis: $n, t, d, \theta, \eth, s,$ and z. Notice that these sounds form a wall that is parallel to the labial wall. When $[n]$ is contrasted to $[\eta]$, $[d]$ to $[g]$, $[t]$ to $[k]$, $[\eth]$ to $[d\mathsf{z}]$, $[\theta]$ to $[t\int]$, $[z]$ to $[\mathsf{z}]$, and $[s]$ to $[\int]$, the importance of tongue placement is highlighted (see Figure 3). The $\eta, g, k,$ $d, t\int, \mathsf{z},$ and $\int$, all, involve the use of the back of the tongue. The three walls—a labial wall, a front lingual wall, and a back lingual wall—constitute

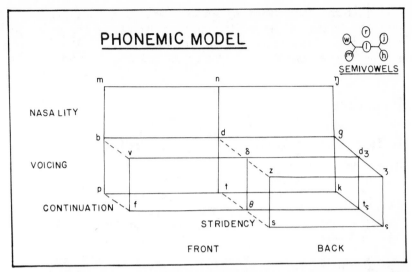

FIGURE 3. A graphic representation of the organization of the consonants and semi-vowels using six distinctive features. Each of the lines that connect the sounds represents one of the features. Sound-pair comparisons are made by noting number and type of features that must be traversed to go from one sound to another, i.e., city-block model.

the major place of articulation dimension. This is a representation of the three-point place of articulation scheme mentioned earlier.

Our third dimension is portrayed in perspective. At the back of the model, you will notice nine stop/nasal sounds: m, n, ŋ, b, d, g, p, t, and k (see Figure 3). These sounds are sometimes referred to as the back-nine system. Relative to the remaining sounds, these nine are interrupted. The remaining sounds are continued. Coming toward you, you will notice six continued sounds: v, f, θ, ð, tʃ, and dʒ. The [b/v] line; the [p/f] line, the [d/ ð] line, the [t/θ] line, the [k/tʃ] line, and the [g/dʒ] line represent the continued/interrupted distinctive feature. Closest to you are the sibilants: s, z, ʃ , and ʒ. These four sounds are continued, but they are also strident to the ear. The [θ/s], the [ð/z], the [tʃ / ʃ], and the [dʒ / ʒ] lines represent the strident/mellow distinctive feature. If you will pronounce 's' to yourself, [s], followed by voiceless 'th,' [θ], you will notice that 's' is much sharper to the ear than the 'th.' All the sibilant sounds share this property. Sibilant sounds are produced by forcing air through an unobstructed dental 'fence.' This results in a great deal of random turbulence. Frequency and intensity characteristics vary greatly making the resulting sound unpleasant to the ear. When the dental 'fence' is obstructed by the tongue or lip, the amount of random turbulence is reduced. This latter condition is perceived as more 'mellow' in character.

If you count all the lines on the model that connect the 19 sounds, you will notice that there are 33 pure feature (minimal) contrasts. Sounds that are separated by more than one line are nonminimal contrasts. The exercises that follow were developed to familiarize you with how the model may be used clinically.

Exercises

1. Isolating the Real Articulation Problem:

Many times it is beneficial in the clinic to know exactly what a sound substitution means. This exercise is designed to help you use the model to determine what sound property is in error. Your task is to determine what *type of feature* is in error when the following sounds are confused. Refer to Figure 3 and locate the two sounds in question. Using the model, locate the defective feature.[2]

    a. [m] and [n]
    b. [t] and [k]
    c. [b] and [v]
    d. [tʃ] and [ʃ]
    e. [ŋ] and [g]
    f. [ʃ] and [ʒ]

2. Evaluating the Severity of a Substitution:

The phonemic model may also be used to compare one sound substitution with another. By counting the number of lines that separate two sounds on the model, the therapist can determine how many features are in error. This exercise is designed to help you determine the *number of features* in error. Refer to Figure 3, locate the two sounds in question, and count the number of lines (features) that separate the following sounds.

    a. [m] and [p]
    b. [θ] and [m]
    c. [m] and [t]
    d. [m] and [ʃ]
    e. [m] and [m]
    f. [ʒ] and [m]

3. Grouping Children for Therapy:

At one time, we used to group children in therapy on the basis of the particular sounds that were in error. In this exercise your task is to evaluate the

---

[2]The answers to the exercises may be found at the end of the chapter.

sound substitution patterns of two therapy groups. The children in Group #1 have the same error sound. The children in Group #2 have different error sounds. Using your ability to determine the type of feature in error (from Exercise 1), compare the two groups.

(a)   Which of the two groups is better organized when you consider the source of confusion, i.e., feature errors?

Group #1	Group #2
Child A– [b/d]	Child F– [m/n]
B– [n/d]	G– [d/b]
C– [g/d]	H– [v/ð]
D– [ð/d]	I– [p/t]
E– [t/d]	J– [f/θ]

Using your ability to determine the number of features in error (from Exercise 2), compare the next two groups. Please answer the following question:

(b)   Which of the two groups is better organized when you consider the severity of the problem, i.e., the average number of features missed by the group?

Group #3	Group #4
Child K– [m/d]	Child P– [m/n]
L– [s/d]	Q– [d/b]
M– [f/d]	R– [v/ð]
N– [t/d]	S– [p/t]
O– [b/d]	T– [f/θ]

If you have worked through the foregoing examples, you will have noticed that grouping children on the basis of the sound in error is not necessarily the best clinical decision. In Exercise 3a, note that the sound-based group (Group #1) has five different problems. Child A does not distinguish the difference between the lips and the tongue. Child B does not understand the importance of velar positioning. Child C does not know the difference between the front and back of the tongue. Child D does not understand the importance of the length of the gesture. The last child E does not understand the implications of the presence or absence of laryngeal activity. On the other hand, Group #2, with five different defective sounds, ([n], [b], [ð], [t], [θ]), is homogeneously based because each child confuses the lips and the tongue. It should be much easier to develop a clinical program for Group #2. All the children in this group have the same type of problem.

From Exercise 3b, it can be noted that the sound-based group (Group #3) varies a great deal in terms of severity. Child N and child O are missing single features in terms of their approximations. Child K has two features missing. Child L and child M are missing three features in terms of their approximations. The latter two children have much more to learn than former children who are missing single features. Group #4, the feature-based group, not only has the same feature to learn, but it is at the same severity level. Each of the children have a single feature in error, the mildest error.

As can be seen from this exercise, a feature-based clinical group can be made more homogeneous than a speech-sound based group. Using features the therapist can isolate the precise therapeutic goal and develop groups that have similar skills and/or deficits.

4. Creating Minimal-Pair Words

At this point, it may be beneficial to pause and try to compose some minimal-pair words.[3] If you were trying to teach the child the importance of the front versus the back of the tongue, what words could be used with:

(a)	'dough' - ' ? '		(d)	'cold'	- ' ? '
(b)	'wing' - ' ? '		(e)	'she'	- ' ? '
(c)	'thief' - ' ? '		(f)	'ten'	- ' ? '

If you have difficulty with this exercise, locate the sound underlined on the phonemic model (Figure 3). The next thing is to locate the desired sound property or distinctive feature. In this example, the feature is the front versus back tongue contrast. There are seven lines directly above the word 'BACK.' Notice that the appropriate line, that which represents the front-versus-back-place tongue contrast, connects [d] to [g]. Therefore, the contrasting word must begin with the [g] and rhyme with 'dough,' i.e., 'go'–[go]. In short, locate the sound, locate the feature, determine the appropriate contrasting phoneme, and develop the word.

To complete this exercise, try the following features and words. Only two examples for each feature will be necessary. Once the nature of the operation is mastered, the task becomes quite simple.

Labial/Lingual (FRONT)
    (g) 'me'   - ' ? '　　　　　　(h) 'bow'   - ' ? '
Voiced/Voiceless (VOICING)
    (i) 'Sue'   - ' ? '　　　　　　(j) 'gold'   - ' ? '
Continued/Interrupted (CONTINUATION)
    (k) 'V'   - ' ? '　　　　　　(l) 'tree'   - ' ? '
Nasal/Non–Nasal (NASALITY)
    (m) 'bee'   - ' ? '　　　　　　(n) 'knee'   - ' ? '
Strident/Mellow (STRIDENCY)
    (o) 'thumb' - ' ? '　　　　　　(p) 'sheep' - ' ? '

---

[3] It is understood that minimal-pair words, for clinical purposes, are graphically represented. Before they are drawn, however, they must be formulated. Notice that example (a) could just as well have been the word "doe."

Roman Jakobson and the System

Roman Jakobson, the man who developed the distinctive feature concept, has emphasized that the system is the most important aspect of phonological study. Speech sounds and features are only significant in reference to the system in which they exist. By implication, speech therapy at the articulatory level is a process of constructing a system as you see represented in Figure 3. In a later part of this presentation, we will look at how this system evolves in a majority of children. But before we get to that, it would be helpful to discuss how distinctive features are taught, using minimal-pair words.

Teaching Distinctive Features

The training of distinctive features is broken down into two major phases: a preparation phase and a presentation phase (see Figure 4).

In the previous discussion, we have begun to lay the foundation for the preparation phase. We will return to Part A in a later part of the presentation. For now, we will concentrate on Part B—the presentation and training of minimal-pairs.

Once a distinctive feature (voicing, etc.), a sound-pair context (t/d, k/g, etc.), and the particular words ("ten"/"den," "tot"/"dot," etc.) have been selected, and the minimal-pair cards have been constructed, the therapist can begin distinctive feature training. There are four major steps in the presentation phase: (1) discussion of the particular words, (2) receptive testing and training, if necessary, (3) productive training, (4) carry-over training.

Step #1: Discussion of Words

In the first step, it is important to determine if the child understands the words you have selected. At times, words will be selected that are not appropriate in terms of the child's vocabulary level. At other times, the picture may not mean the same thing to the child as it does to you. For instance, a picture of a boy's face may be used to represent the word 'boy,' 'face,' 'Bobby,' 'Ted,' 'head,' etc. It is important to orient the child to just what he or she is expected to say. In this step, the basic question is "Does the child know the ideas I am working with?" If the child does not understand the ideas that underlie the phonetic/phonemic[4] contrast, the child will have to be taught the

---

[4] The term phonetic/phonemic is used to imply a psycholinguistic phenomena, over and above a simple sound gesture. A phoneme and its subcomponent features is viewed as a socially defined set of acoustic parameters which are physiologically produced and psychologically interpreted in order to transfer ideas from one individual to another. The term 'phonetic' implies the physio-acoustic parameters. The term 'phonemic' implies the psycho-social parameters. (See Blache, 1978a, pp. 20–25.) The combined term 'phonetic/phonemic' is used to represent the complexity of the process in question.

MINIMAL WORD-PAIRS ORIENTATION

A. PREPARATION PHASE:

1. DIAGNOSIS — Evaluate for etiologies and symptoms

2. SYSTEM SELECTION — "Stop-Nasals"(velars)

3. FEATURE SELECTION — Back-Place ±

4. SOUND-PAIR SELECTION — [t/k] [d/g]

5. WORD-PAIR SELECTION — "tea/key; tape/cape; etc."—"bat/back; pit/pick"

6. CARD CONSTRUCTION — a^1 a^2 b^1 b^2

B. PRESENTATION PHASE:

1. DISCUSSION OF WORDS — Does the child have the ideas?

2. RECEPTIVE TRAINING — Therapist pronounces / Child gestures

3. PRODUCTIVE TRAINING — Child pronounces / Therapist gestures

4. CARRY-OVER TRAINING — Longer responses and home training

FIGURE 4. A graphic representation of the strategy used to organize a minimal word-pairs training program. This model is used to chart therapeutic progress and revise programs where failure is encountered (a = selection of new prevocalic contrasts; b = selection of new postvocalic contrasts and/or new sound-pairs; c = selection of new features; d = selection of new sound systems or developmental stages).

concepts in question before they can be labeled. Usually, it is more convenient to choose another word-pair. For instance, a child who is unfamiliar with the alphabet will have difficulty with "T"/"key." Using "tea"/"key" holds the feature (BACK PLACE), sound-pair (t/k), and phonetic shape $[ti]/[ki]$ constant, and shifts the semantic referrent.

As a rule, change the picture before the phonetic shape, i.e., semantic referrent. If the phonetic shape must be changed, hold the feature (BACK PLACE) and sound-pair (t/k) constant, and vary the rhyming element, i.e., "told"/"cold," "ten"/"Ken," etc. If no success is found with (t/k), hold the feature (BACK PLACE) constant and vary the sound-pair, i.e., $[d/g]$—BACK PLACE, $[n/\eta]$—BACK PLACE, etc. If the feature is the source of the problem, change the feature in reference to the appropriate developmental system. If you will refer to Figure 4, this procedure represents a shift from A-6 to A-5, A-5 to A-4, A-4 to A-3, A-3 to A-2. Finally, it is also possible that the problem is not simply a deficit in learning, but is organically based. If so, the child's educational program should be supplemented with socio-medical management.

In our protocol, we simply indicate the topic of discussion and ask the children if they have ever heard the words before. If a child indicates that he/she has heard the words before, we ask a series of either/or questions concerning the pictures, and ask the child to indicate which picture we are referring to. If the child seems to be confused about the ideas actually represented, we choose other words that will teach the same feature with the same sound-pair (see Blache, 1978b; Blache and Parsons, 1980; Blache, Parsons and Humphreys, 1981).

Step #2: Receptive Testing and Training

Once the child indicates that he or she knows the ideas you are talking about, the next task is to determine whether the child can perceive the phonetic feature that is separating the two words. Our research has shown that a significant number of children have adequate hearing, but do not attend to certain sound properties (Blache, DeMaio and Brown-Harding, 1978; Blache and Rodd, 1979). To check for this type of problem, the therapist pronounces the two words, in a random fashion, and asks the child to point to the word that has been said. The therapist then counts the number of consecutive correct responses.

Various criterion levels can be used. A child, by pure chance, will get 5 consecutive correct responses 3 times in 100 trials; 6 correct, 3 times in 200; 7 correct, 8 times in 1000; and 8 correct, 4 times in 1000. The object is to select a level where one is confident that the child's consecutive correct responses are not due to chance, but a true indication of an ability to discriminate between the two words. In our program, we use 6 consecutive correct responses as the criterion. If a child correctly identifies the random production of the two words for 6 consecutive trials, we assume the child is perceiving the feature in question. On occasion, a child gets lucky and we are in error. The success in the following therapeutic stage, however, is dependent upon perceptual feedback. If an error occurs in the following stage, we will return to this stage and retest the word-pair.

Step #3: Production Training

This stage in distinctive feature training is the most exciting. It is the 'moment of truth.' Children are told that they are to act as the teacher. The child is given control of the situation. He or she is instructed to say the words as the teacher. In turn, the therapist will point to the words pronounced. In this fashion, children are permitted to put their verbal skills to the test. The therapist provides visual feedback as to the adequacy of the verbal skills.

When the child is permitted to pronounce the two words, the following can be expected to occur: Most children will say the word they can pronounce effectively, as their first attempt and, in their second attempt, will try to say the alternate word. Due to the feature error, however, they use a pronunciation similar to the first word. The child expects the therapist's finger to move to the second picture. The therapist hears a pronunciation similar to the first word, however, and does not move the finger. This is the 'moment of truth.' The child wanted the therapist's finger to move to the other picture— the therapist's finger did not move. The child's task is to develop an articulatory strategy to get the finger to move to the other picture.

At this point in therapy, the child is highly motivated. Sometimes the child will point to the other picture. The child uses gesture to compensate for the lack of phonetic skill. At other times, the child will tell the therapist that he or she is in error. The therapist asks the child if he/she is trying to say the target word (which is the case). The child answers in the affirmative. The therapist then offers to help the child say the word. Textbooks are full of 'clinical tricks' for eliciting articulatory gestures. Regardless of the clinical device used to elicit the proper gesture, one thing should be kept in mind: the goal of the task is pronouncing words. The clinical cue should be directed at a *word level approximation*. The minimal word-pairs approach is designed to 'weld' the sound gesture to its function—making words different.

It is very helpful throughout this stage to watch the child's line-of-sight. This is an excellent indicator of the child's linguistic intent. The child generally will look at the word he is trying to say, and then watch for your gesture. In very abstract terms, it has been said that language permits man to manipulate reality. The minimal word-pairs approach crystallizes this concept into a game that can be played by children. Ultimately, the child must discover phonetic skills to play phonemic games. Each word-pair stimulates psycholinguistic development by posing a phonetic problem of relevance to the culture's phonemic system. It cannot be expected that each and every permutation of the phonemic system can be trained. The ultimate hope is that children will begin to understand that they are not communicating some words properly. In turn, they are encouraged to experiment with new articulatory concepts (features). The therapist then guides the child to the appropriate concepts through articulatory clues or 'clinical tricks.' Once success has been exhibited, the therapist charts new tasks (different words, different word positions, different sound-pairs) and sets new goals (different features).

Aberrant Approximations.   While it can be very exciting to see children experiment with new articulatory concepts, it requires the active intellectual commitment of the therapist to the process. For instance, a therapist is working with a child who is 'fronting' (using [t] where one would expect [k]). The words "T"/"key" are chosen to teach the importance of raising the back portion of the tongue to the velum. It has been determined that the child knows the respective ideas and can discriminate between the differences in pronunciation. The child is asked to be the teacher and pronounces "T" correctly, i.e., [ti]. The child then attempts to say, "Key." The utterance used is [tʃi]. There is a natural tendency to conclude that the child's approximation was incorrect because the utterance and the target word were not identical. The therapeutic goal, however, was to teach the child to use the back portion of the tongue. If you will refer to Figure 3, you will note that [tʃ] is very similar to [k]. The difference between [t] and [k] is BACK PLACE; the differences between [t] and [tʃ] are BACK PLACE and CONTINUATION. The child's approximation represents the generation of the correct feature, plus an extra one. In this approach, therapists are encouraged to accept these types of approximations and move their fingers. Our experience has shown that children who are not rewarded for phonemic overapproximations tend to become confused and cease to experiment with new articulatory strategies. For this reason, we accept the overapproximation, and at a later point in the program we remove the extra feature. To simplify the decision as to whether an approximation should be reinforcd, we use the rule "reinforce the *feature* not the sound." This, of course, places demands upon the therapist to constantly monitor articulatory shifts and evaluate their appropriateness. A therapist's discrimination skills and knowlede of articulatory phonetics are put to the test. The smile that accompanies the production of the target word does a great deal to compensate for the concentration required.

Step #4: Carry-Over Training

Once the child demonstrates consistent control of the desired feature, work is begun to encourage use of the target words in everyday speech. Emphasis is placed on two objectives. The child is encouraged to use the target word at the end of longer and longer expressions. The child is also encouraged to use the target words in the home situation.

Carry-Over into Connected Speech. Once the child demonstrates that he or she can say the target word, the target word and the distinctive feature 'lure' are put at the end of one-word, two-word, three-word, and four-word expressions. Instead of saying "key" or "T," the child is expected to say, "The key" or "The 'T'." This is followed by "Touch the key/Touch the 'T' " (3-word level); "Point to the key/Point to the 'T' " (4-word level). The goal of the task is to strengthen memory and muscular synthesis. When a child demonstrates an ability to pronounce a word and an inability to use the word in combination with other words, the therapist can expand the therapy program at the two-word level by using the coarticulatory approach of McDonald (1964). The definite article, 'the,' is replaced by other words that will call into play significant coarticulatory combinations. This modification presumes an underlying physiological base for the problem. If, on the other hand, the problem is due to poor auditory memory, we return to the discrimination task at the one-word level. With this modification, the therapist pronounces one of the two words and asks the child to point to the word that has been said. To strengthen auditory memory, however, the child does not see the pictures immediately. A word is pronounced. The therapist waits for a period of time. The two cards are then turned over and the child is asked to identify which word was said. (For a discussion of the use of minimal-pairs with auditory memory see Blache and O'Brien, 1979; Blache, Parsons, and DeMaio, 1977.) It is possible to anticipate problems due to auditory memory span and coarticulatory difficulty. The current approach presumes a learning deficit. If there is specific structural or physiological etiology, it should have been isolated during the initial diagnostic assessment. The test battery used with this approach will be discussed in the last section of this presentation.

Carry-Over into the Home Situation. Our literature is replete with studies demonstrating that some children will learn to speak one way in the clinical situation and another way at home. To avoid problems such as this, we encourage therapists to involve parents in the therapy program. The parents are encouraged to stimulate verbal activity, serve as a receptive audience, and monitor the child's productions. When children demonstrate mastery of particular words, the respective picture is put into a 'Word Book.' The parents are asked to set aside a regular period of family time for word recitation. It is suggested that, following the evening meal, the child is given the opportunity to recite new words learned and old words mastered. The parents are instructed to praise all words correctly pronounced. They are cautioned not to comment on unusual pronunciations, however. The parents are not equipped to determine if a unusual pronunciation represents an improvement or not. When unusual pronunciations are detected, the parents are asked to report the 'problem' at the next clinical visit. At that time, the parents are counseled as to whether a particular pronunciation is to be reinforced or not. At the beginning of each therapy session, the parents are asked how the child is doing at home. At this time, the therapist is monitoring not only the success of the child in the home situation, but the parents' ability to provide the proper support for articulatory development.

Developing Phonemic Strategies

Up to this point, we have looked at the minimal word-pairs approach as if it were restricted to the teaching of a particular distinctive feature in a single context. It cannot be assumed that learning a distinctive feature with just two words will guarantee a complete appreciation of the feature in all communication contexts, however. The child must learn that the particular feature is important in various word contexts, in various word positions, and various sound-pairs contexts. In other words, the minimal word-pairs approach is both a tactic and a strategy. The particular way in which the therapist teaches the distinctive feature with the words and pictures is the tactic. The manner in which the child is taught to generalize the feature to other words, other segmental positions, and other sound-pair contrasts is the strategy. If you will refer to Figure 4, you will notice that the preparation phase involves the development of the therapeutic strategy. Once the therapist determines whether the problem is primarily a learning deficit or an organically based problem (A-1), a program of therapy is designed to rebuild a certain part, or parts, of the phonemic system. If the problem is due to incomplete or retarded phonemic growth, the level of development will be determined and a normal remedial strategy will be established. If the problem is due to an historical or sustaining etiological agent, a management program will be developed to supplement the educational program.

In this approach, the educational program entails a strategic hierarchy. Word pairs are used to teach the importance of sound-pair contrasts. Sound-pair contrasts are used to teach the importance of distinctive features. Distinctive features are used to teach the importance of the phonemic system. The ultimate goal of putting two words in opposition is to rebuild an undeveloped or defective phonemic system. Therapeutic planning begins with the part or parts of the system to be rebuilt. This type of strategy is *paradigmatic* in character. The therapist is trying to establish a phonemic potential that can be used at any moment in time. Hence, the term 'paradigmatic.' At the same time, the therapist is developing the use of this potential, sequentially, over time. When the therapist varies the position of contrast, and increases the length of the utterance (segments per words or words per phrase), we say that the therapist is pursuing a *syntagmatic* strategy. Currently, much is being written concerning the development of syntagmatic programs. The remaining portion of this presentation will concentrate on paradigmatic programming.

The Minimal Word-Pairs Tactic

The philosophy that led to the tactical nature of the minimal word-pair was quite simple. It was felt that no one therapeutic program could be powerful enough to correct the variety of ways in which the sound system is mal-formed, i.e., symptom patterns. In addition to this, it was felt that no one treatment program is powerful enough to respond to the many etiological agents that may cause the speech sound system to be malformed. At best, it was thought that the treatment program should provide a skeletal structure flexible enough to meet the variety of symptomatic and etiological patterns possible. At the same time, the approach chosen was to be finite enough to crystallize the essence of the phonetic/phonemic code and the communi-cation act, i.e., transmitting an idea from one individual to another through a mutually agreeable code.

Figure 4 represents an abstraction of the therapeutic process. Although not directly indicated, it is understood that modifications will always occur. It is assumed that children vary greatly and must be treated as individuals. The sequence of steps during preparation and presentation is designed to organize a variety of therapeutic approaches into a comprehensive proce-dure for attacking problems. Clinicians who have used progressive approx-imation, auditory discrimination training, auditory memory techniques, associative learning strategies, play therapy, motokinesthetic cues, or other approaches are encouraged to view the therapeutic model (Figure 4) as a method of organizing their techniques into a flexible, linguistically-based treatment program. While learning distinctive features is often self-rein-forcing, at times the therapist will have to introduce reinforcement programs to keep the child motivated. The minimal word-pairs tactic is designed to encourage the child to develop carry-over as soon as possible and encourage the therapist to attend to the specific goal behavior. The minimal word-pairs strategy is designed to provide a frame comprehensive enough to integrate traditional therapeutic technique and modern linguistic theory.

Selecting Distinctive Features

The rationale that was used to develop our distinctive feature organization is quite complex and cannot be discussed in any detail here. For those interested, refer to *The Acquisition of Distinctive Features* (Blache, 1978a). In this presentation, I will outline the patterns of distinctive feature acquisition briefly. Following this, I will demonstrate one method of selecting specific features for therapy.

The Six Phonemic Stages

Using the developmental studies of Templin (1957), Poole (1934), and Wellman (1931), the phonological acquisition frame of Jakobson (1941; 1968), and the results of extensive psychoacoustic research from 1948 to 1968, we have concluded that children's phonemic development may be determined to be in one of six basic stages of systematic growth. We have labeled these stages: (1) the primitive, (2) the vocalic, (3) the stop-nasal, (4) the semivowel, (5) the continuant, and (6) the sibilant stage (see Figure 5).

SUBSYSTEMS

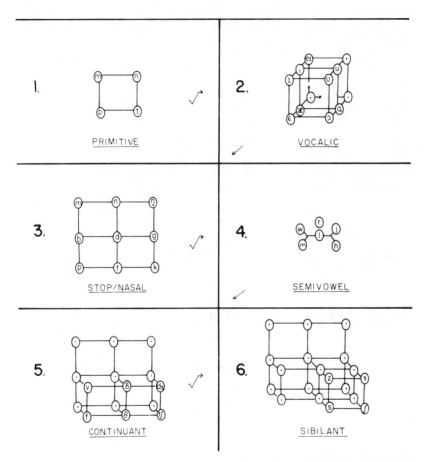

FIGURE 5. A model of the six basic stages of phonemic growth. Stages 1, 3, 5, and 6 represent expansion of the consonantal system; Stage 2, the organization of the vowel system; Stage 4, the organization of the semivowel system.

During the period from 18 months to 8 years of age, the child is viewed as developing a mastery of vowels, consonants, and sound elements that contain both consonantal and vocalic characteristics, and word boundary markers. The six stages represent consolidation, expansion, and reorganization of sound properties necessary to produce syllable shapes that can be differentiated. At its zenith, phonemic growth is seen as the development of a well-organized consonant system, a well-organized semivowel system, and an ability to recognize word, phrase, and sentence shapes. Stages 1–primitive, 3–stop/nasal, 5–continuant, and 6–sibilant represent a complex adjustment pattern necessary for the organization of consonants. Stage 2–vocalic marks the organization of vowels; the first system to be put under complete control. Stage 4–semivowel represents an almost complete organization of sound elements necessary to extend CV⁻ and ⁻VC syllable patterns to CCV⁻ and ⁻VCC syllable patterns. In all, six stages are used to represent the development of three major systems (see Figure 6).

MAJOR SYSTEMS

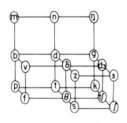

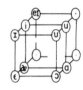

CONSONANTS   SEMIVOWELS   VOWELS

FIGURE 6. A model of the three basic systems used to sequence phonetic/phonemic shapes and transform them into syllable structures. Whereas Figure 5 represents paradigmatic expansion, the current figure represents the basic pattern underlying syntagmatic expansion.

The systems, in turn, are used to generate segmental length. Because distinctive feature theory was originally framed to explain the evolution of the child's paradigmatic development, I will restrict the discussion to the evolution of these three sound systems, rather than their sequential use. It should not be assumed, however, that there is an inherent reason why syntagmatic development cannot be described through a distinctive feature approach.

Stage #1: The Primitive System

By approximately 18 months of age, the child is expected to have been exposed to an extensive amount of linguistic stimulation. The child should have an awareness of the presence of phonetic properties of the language (see Cairns and Butterfield, 1978). Too, the child should have developed a certain amount of control of the articulatory structures necessary for phonemic utterances (see Oller, 1978; cf. Blache, 1978a, pp. 89–102; Stark, 1978, pp. 131–140). This growing capacity to produce phonemic utterances is paralleled by a growing social awareness and a desire to communicate in an adult fashion. Sometime between 9 months and 24 months, the child will try to produce a vocal utterance to transfer meaning. At this time, the child will have had to develop an understanding of the linguistic importance of basic consonantal and vocalic characteristics in order to formulate a simple syllable shape to carry meaning. The child should be able to differentiate utterances that tend to be brief, closed, and anterior in the vocal track (consonant-like) from those that are much longer, open, and laryngeal in locus (vowel-like). Using this somewhat crude understanding, in conjunction with the desire to 'say a word,' it is expected that the child will produce a syllable shape that contrasts brief, relatively weak, aperiodic noise with a prolonged, relatively intense, periodic vowel tone. From this understanding of the motor-acoustic parameters of the syllable, the child will begin a process in which the vague CV–shape is differentiated into a meaningful phonemic system.

In the primitive stage, the child is expected to develop command of two distinctive features that serve as the foundation of the consonantal system (see Figure 7). At this level of development, the child is perceived as mastering the implications that result from categorizing sounds with both the nasal/non-nasal feature and the labial/lingual feature. Whereas, in the first year to a year-and-a-half of life, the child has experimented with phonetic

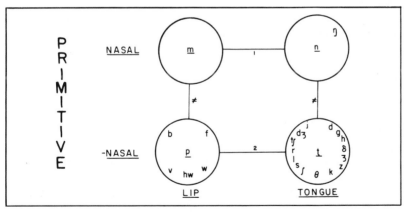

FIGURE 7. A model of the organization of the earliest developing consonantal system. The lines represent the features that have become distinctive. Within each circle are the permissible free varying elements, i.e., distinctive feature errors or sound substitution processes. The most probable adult utterance is underlined. The circle represents the child's infanteme.

properties, the child must now organize those properties into a well-organized, operational system. This rapid phoneme generator must coordinate the child's phonetic potential and interface with the child's semantic intent. Figure 7 represents a model of the results of distinctive feature decisions. At this stage, the child produces utterances of four types: a nasal, labial utterance (usually in the form of [m]), a nasal, lingual utterance (usually in the form of [n]), a non-nasal, labial utterance (usually in the form of [p]), and a non-nasal, lingual utterance (usually in the form of [t]). Although somewhat crude, these four utterances are fully phonemic in character. The child uses the utterances to convey differential meaning.

Jakobson (1968) has noted that during this period children tend to produce reduplicated structures of the baby-talk sort: "mama," "papa," "nana," "tata." This rudimentary four-word vocabulary, centering on the infantile labels for family members, household objects, pets, etc., serves as the first form of meaningful communication. As a child attempts to expand his or her meaningful vocabulary, pressure will be brought to bear to develop more significant sound properties and more sophisticated syllable shapes. The motor-acoustic information that has been stored from birth is now being organized phonemically and put under active control in order to communicate.

If a child could respond to an articulation test at this age, we would anticipate a diagnosis of a severe, multiple-articulation problem. As can be noted in the model of this stage in Figure 7, many sounds in the lingual, non-nasal class are confused with one another. Likewise, the labial, non-nasal class contains sound utterances in free variation with each other. The child's phonemic knowledge, at this stage, is represented by the lines that separate the utterances. The child is aware of the nasal/non-nasal ($\neq$ / $\neq$) and the labial/lingual (1, 2) contrasts. The sounds which have the highest probability of being used to represent the infanteme[5] are underlined and centered. However, any sound utterance within a circle could be used (c.f. Weiner, 1981). The only requirement necessary for the attainment of this stage is for the child not to confuse nasal sounds with non-nasal sounds and labial sounds with lingual sounds.

Stage #2: The Vowels

By three years of age, most children have generally mastered the subtle differences in vocalic production. The refined shifts in lingual posture which result in consistent production of recognizable formant patterns are phenomena worthy of amazement. We have retained the universal developmental frame outlined by Jakobson (1968) and confirmed by Leopold (1971).

---

[5] An *infanteme* is defined as a set of concurrent sound properties which serve to differentiate words of unlike meaning *in the language of the child*. The term is taken from Haas (1963) and the definition is an extension of Jakobson's (1962) definition of the phoneme.

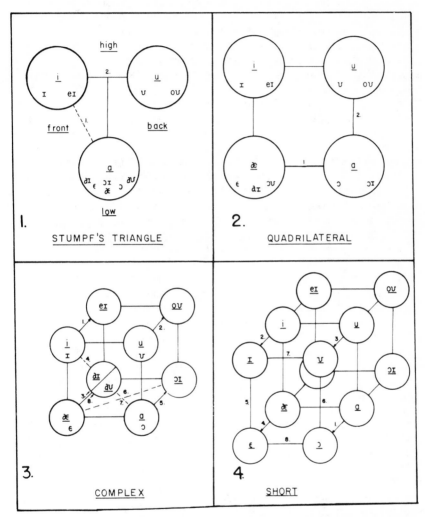

FIGURE 8. A model of the four substages of vocalic expansion and organization. (Note restriction in permissible free variation as the child learns more and more distinctive features.)

In their view, the vowel system evolves through a process in which the child first learns the importance of raising the rear portion of the tongue. This movement tends to shift the acoustic energy, generally associated with [a], out of its central locus. As soon as this effect has been mastered, the child learns the importance of moving in an anterior-posterior direction. This form of movement causes the second formant to raise or lower in frequency. In this manner, the child probes the external limits of the vowel triangle from a physiological and acoustical perspective (see Figure 8–#1). With this motor-acoustic foundation established, we have interpolated an expansion appropriate for our language.

Research has shown that vowels are not produced in a truly triangular fashion. Physiologically, vowel postures tend to be limited in the form of a quadrilateral. This phenomena is represented in Figure 8 (#2). This substage represents a refinement in the low vowel utterances. At this level of development, the child has four vowel-like infantemes: a high-front utterance, a low-front utterance, a high-back utterance, and a low-back utterance. As can be noted in the model, many vowels are still being confused with each other—but high vowels will not be confused with low vowels and front vowels will not be confused with back vowels.

Once a child has organized the basic motor-acoustic frame of the vowels, it is expected that he or she will be able to contend with those phonemes that move within the frame, i.e., the diphthongs. We have labeled this distinctive feature complex/noncomplex (see Figure 8–#3). At this substage, the child is not expected to confuse the four standard motor-acoustic postures with the utterances that tend to move within the frame. As a final step in vocalic expansion, the child learns to control and generate vowel-like utterances, which are short in character. These utterances are acoustically similar to the four primary vowels in terms of frequency, but tend to be produced in a shorter fashion (see Figure 8–#4). As can be noted from the model, the acquisition of the two features complex/noncomplex and short/normal creates a dimension that ultimately relates to the duration of the vowel. Ultimately, the vowel system is seen as a structure that regulates timing characteristics and frequency standards. All of this development is completed by the third year of life. The development of the vowel system and its subsequent and/or simultaneous integration with the consonants creates great linguistic potential to generate common two syllable words. With this skill, however, comes additional stress to extend the consonantal system of the previous stage to produce more phonetically sophisticated segmental expressions. With growth in semantic intent, the child must develop utterances more varied in type and segmental order.

Stage #3: The Stop/Nasal System

By four years of age, it is expected that the average child will have introduced two new distinctive features into his or her phonemic repertoire. These two features represent a major extension of the primitive consonantal system developed in stage #1 (see Figure 9).

In this stage, a child refines his or her understanding of manner and place of articulation by developing a more precise definition of nasal/non-nasal and labial/lingual. I will comment on each extension separately.

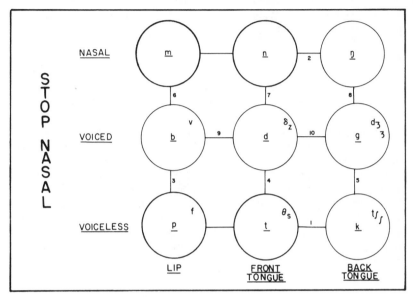

FIGURE 9. A model of the expansion of the primitive consonantal system into the stop/nasal system. (Note the addition of velarization and the refinement of nasal/non-nasal by means of the voiced/voiceless feature.)

Place of Articulation. In its earliest stage, place of articulation is understood, in a vague sense, as a labial utterance contrasted with an utterance made by the tongue. In the current stage, the lingual utterance is refined into an anterior lingual utterance versus a posterior lingual utterance. The establishment of the lingual contrast expresses itself as greater control over the acoustic parameters associated with velar sounds. It is expected that consonant-vowel transitions will stabilize and the aperiodic turbulence associated with prevocalic plosives will be differentiated from labial and lingua-alveolar sounds. Ultimately, the stops and nasals are categorized into a three-point place of articulation scheme. (For similar findings see Blache, 1979; Blache and Martin, 1977; Miller and Nicely, 1955; Olmsted, 1971; Wicklegren, 1966.) This place of articulation scheme will be retained throughout all subsequent consonantal development.

Manner of Articulation. In stage #1, nasality was established through the development of an understanding of the implications of closing the velopharyngeal port. In the present stage, the child will differentiate between two types of utterances produced with a closed port, i.e., voiced versus voiceless (see Figure 9). In the primitive stage, voiceless stops are expected to be used in opposition to nasals for they lack the voicing component that is present with nasals. In stage #3, the $[b]$–, $[d]$–, and $[g]$–like gestures are differentiated from their voiceless counterparts on the basis of the presence or absence of laryngeal activity. At the same time, these utterances are contrasted with their nasal counterparts on the basis of the nature of their spectral and timing differences.

Implications. This stage represents the suppression of the 'fronting' process in which anterior lingual sounds are used to replace posterior lingual sounds. As will be noted from the infantemic configurations from Figure 9, the 'stopping' process should still manifest itself as a normal way of marking continuants and sibilants. At the same time, phonological processes associated with voicing or devoicing should tend to diminish. The child, however, is learning to use longer and longer segmental combinations. It would seem unwise to assume that laryngeal-based processes will be totally eliminated. At this stage, we feel that the child can differentiate between nine basic consonantal utterances: nasal-labial, voiced-labial, voiceless-labial, nasal-(front) lingual, voiced-(front) lingual, voiceless-(front) lingual, nasal-(back) lingual, voiced-(back) lingual, and voiceless-(back) lingual. While several adult utterances may be used to represent such phonemic skills, $[m]$, $[b]$, $[p]$, $[n]$, $[d]$, $[t]$, $[\theta]$, $[g]$, and $[k]$ are considered to be the most probable to become stable.

Stage #4: The Semivowel System

After the child has established velars and voiced stops into a nine-category consonantal system, we anticipate a stabilization of the semivowels. By the latter part of the fourth year, the average child is assumed to have discovered that some adult utterances behave very much like consonants as well as vowels. These utterances are vowel-like in tone but variable and rapid enough to mark the onset or termination of vowels.

These utterances, which have both consonantal and vowel characteristics, are organized into a three-point place of articulation scheme similar to the stop/nasals (see Figure 10). As this system unfolds, the labial semivowel $[w/hw]$, which to this date is often used to replace a majority of semivowels, is differentiated along labial/lingual lines followed by a front versus back tongue contrast. As the situation demands, the voiced/voiceless characteristics will be integrated into the system. Finally, the $[r]$ will be appended to the semivowels with all its acoustic subtleties (see Kantner and West, 1960, pp. 168–178).

Phonological processes associated with such terms as 'liquidization,' 'gliding,' and 'centralizing' should be in remission in this stage. At the same time, the stability of the semivowels tends to create more strength with certain

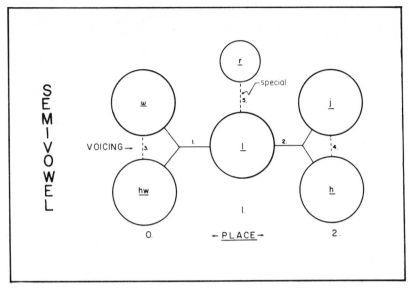

FIGURE 10. A model of the semivowel system. The lines represent the features that have become distinctive. The arabic numerals above each line represent the order of expansion of the system and the tentative order for minimal word-pairs programming.

clusters. Phonological processes associated with [l] and [r] cluster reductions should also be in remission (c.f. Ingram, 1976, pp. 32–34).

Stage #5: The Continuant System

By the latter part of the fifth year, the average child is expected to have grasped the importance of, and begun to control, the duration of the consonantal signal. In this stage, the child has developed an ability to prolong an aperiodic utterance, and has integrated the linguistic importance of such an articulatory device into the phonemic system (see Figure 11).

The introduction of the continuation feature is a complicated phenomenon. While the concept may be one easily grasped, the full implications of the feature are difficult to contend with. Before this stage the child has had control over nine consonantal utterances. The continuant/interrupted feature will increase the stop/nasal system by almost 50 percent. As the child begins to use utterances longer in duration, he or she will have to differentiate among the new utterances, using the place and manner features from the previous sound system. Not only will the child have to produce continuants, but he must also differentiate among these continuants using voiced/voiceless characteristics and labial–(front) lingual and (back) lingual. While previous stages have been devoted primarily to the acquisition of new distinctive features, this stage is devoted to generalization of previously learned information.

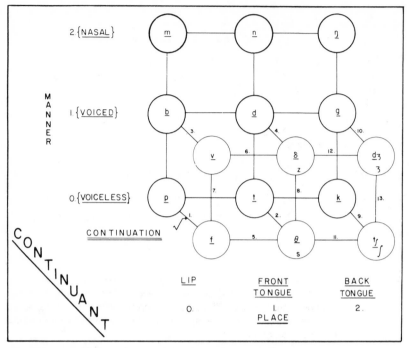

FIGURE 11. A model of the expansion of the stop/nasal system into the continuant system. The lines with arabic numerals represent the new sound-pair contrasts which have become distinctive. These numerals represent the tentative order for programming. (Note free variation.)

At the same time, new subtleties are introduced. The acoustic manifestation of place and manner characteristics changes in the continuant class. The acoustic characteristics associated with brief utterances must be re-evaluated as they are, as some call it, 'smeared' (see Sommerstein, 1977). The child must contend with new acoustic standards and integrate the results into the phonemic system. The end-product is an infantemic repertoire that closely approximates the adult model. At completion, few articulatory errors are observed by laymen. The trained phonetician will note a developmentally based 'lisp' and poor control over sibilants in general.

It is interesting to note that the various stages presented have their equivalents in clinical terms. A child who does not complete the development of the semivowel system is typicaly called a 'laller.' A child with incomplete development at the onset of the continuant stage is referred to as 'a baby talker;' at the end of this stage, 'a lisper.' Distinctive feature theory has, at times, been viewed as a set of mystical terms for strange phenomena. Upon close examination, the theory is a simplification of a complicated process that may take years to develop. Up to this point, we have examined what it means for the child to discover the importance of the larynx, the velum, the lips, the teeth, and the tongue. The problem has been to coordinate this physiological structure into a consistent acoustic generator recognizable to adults.

Stage #6: The Sibilant System

The last stage of development represents a refinement in the continuant class. Those sounds which require unobstructed dental airflow are contrasted to their obstructed counterparts (see Figure 12).

The technical term for this distinctive feature is 'strident/mellow.' The sibilants, as a class, require the teeth to be unobstructed in order for a great deal of turbulence to occur. This results in a sound which varies greatly in terms of frequency and intensity components. When the tongue obstructs the airflow, the sound becomes less variable in terms of frequency and intensity.

It can be noted that the introduction of this feature requires the generalization of earlier learned features—as did the introduction of continuation.

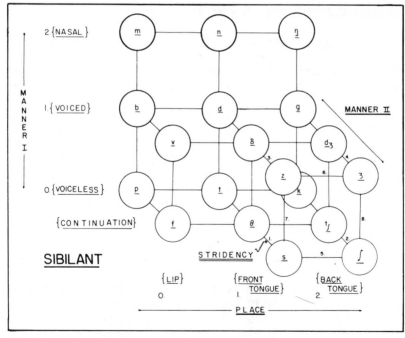

FIGURE 12. A model of the expansion of the continuant system into the sibilant system. This is equivalent to the adult system. (Note the order of development and tentative order for programming.)

With the sibilants, the child separates the sounds with voiced/voiceless and front/back tongue contrasts. Failure to distinguish the importance of front-versus-back tongue placement results in the common lateral lisp. Failure to distinguish the importance of stridency results in the interdental lisp.

Summary

If you will compare Figure 12 to Figure 3, you will note that they are equivalent. I have, in the last section, described our conception of how the phonemic model grows from 18 months to its adult form. We anticipate that the sibilants will be stabilized between the sixth and the eighth year. Note, too, that this expansion is only one aspect of a larger system that also includes vowels (see Figure 6). In all, I have sketched a general frame of feature acquisition. I have pointed out those adult sounds that tend to be used to represent the features. I have cautioned, however, that features are being acquired, not sounds. At the same time, I have emphasized that the features are learned in reference to patterns called "systems." It is upon these systems that therapy is based.

Choosing Where to Begin

In order to select a distinctive feature for training with the minimal word-pair-approach, I suggest a strategy that can be applied in the typical clinical setting. This strategy is not the most sophisticated, but it is practical. To begin developing a minimal word-pairs program, I would suggest the procedure as follows:

> 1. Administer an articulation test that contains the sounds [m n ŋ p t k b d g w l r j h f v θ ðtʃ dʒ s z ʃ ʒ] in enough contexts to determine if each sound is adequate for speech. If a very young age group is the subject, vowels should also be tested. Note the defective sounds.
> 2. Look at the respective sounds in the stop/nasal, semivowel, continuant, and sibilant systems in developmental order. If two or more sounds are in error, begin in that system, i.e., the earliest developing system. It should be remembered that this is not a training program but a stimulation program. The phonemic system is stimulated to grow at the earliest point expressing organizational problems.
> 3. Refer to the respective models of the system as presented in Figure 9, 10, 11, and 12. This is the system to be stimulated.
> 4. Using the defective sounds as a reference, note all connecting lines that touch the defective sound, or sounds. Each of these lines has a number associated with it. These numbers represent a provisional order for teaching the sound-pair contrasts. Make a list of all sound-pair contrasts and note the features they represent.

5. Once you have the list of sound-pairs and features to be taught, formulate minimal pairs at the word level that are appropriate to the respective child. Note the stabilization of each distinctive feature on the model as sound-pair contrasts are acquired.

6. If difficulties are experienced with the prescribed order, change the therapeutic goal in reference to the model. The models are a means of helping you visualize the therapeutic strategy.

Differential Diagnosis

The therapeutic program that has been described is focused upon phonemic problems associated with deficient learning. it is important to adapt the program if etiological agents are present. The test battery I use is presented in Appendix A. We have assumed that it is essential to examine both the environment and the child to determine if there is an identifiable cause for the problem. We suggest that consideration be given to the possibility of a second language in the home, a possible regional dialect, or an unusual speech model in the home. In particular, we are concerned about the existence of family members who interpret for the child in question. It is assumed that each child will have an audiometric screening test and a thorough examination of the structure and function of the articulators. Consideration is also given to the level of motivation and the inherent intellectual capacity for developing communication skills. If problems are found with the child's intellect, emotions, anatomy and physiology, audition, or home situation, a management program is introduced to treat the problem at all levels. In addition to this, I have found it very profitable to check not only the child's ability to produce speech sounds, but his or her ability to remember and discriminate among them. This procedure often lets us anticipate areas of future difficulty with the minimal word-pairs.

Final Comments

In all, I am sure that I have left much unsaid. I am aware that more needs to be done to the minimal word-pairs orientation to refine it as a therapeutic model. We are pleased, however, with the results of our initial testing of the approach. I hope that you will find it to be a plausible alternative to a speech sound approach.

The author would like to thank the New Hampshire Speech and Hearing Association, who first requested the development of the workshop program which forms the basis of this chapter. In addition, the author would like to express his gratitude to Central Michigan University for including this presentation in such a prestigious forum. Finally, thanks are expressed to Drs. Joann Fokes and Sadanand Singh without whose encouragement the current presentation and *The Acquisition of Distinctive Features* would have languished.

Answers to Exercises

1. Type of Features in error:
   - a. labial/lingual
   - b. front/back lingual
   - c. continued/interrupted
   - d. strident/mellow
   - e. nasal/non-nasal
   - f. voiced/voiceless

2. Number of Features in error:
   - a. 2 features
   - b. 4 features
   - c. 3 features
   - d. 6 features
   - e. 0 features
   - f. 5 features

3. *Clinical Grouping:*
   (a) by type of problem—Group #2 is better organized. Each child in this group confuses the lips and the tongue.

Group #1	*Group #2*
A. labial/lingual	F. labial/lingual
B. nasal/non-nasal	G. labial/lingual
C. front/back lingual	H. labial/lingual
D. continued/interrupted	I. labial/lingual
E. voiced/voiceless	J. labial/lingual

   (b) by severity of the problem—Group #4 is better organized. Each child has one feature in error. In Group #3 there is great variability.

Group #3	*Group #4*
K. 2 features	P. 1 feature
L. 3 features	Q. 1 feature
M. 3 features	R. 1 feature
N. 1 feature	S. 1 feature
O. 1 feature	T. 1 feature

4. *Minimal Word-Pair Construction:*

   Front/Back Lingual
   - (a) "go"
   - (b) "wig"
   - (c) "chief"
   - (d) "told"
   - (e) "see," "C," "sea"
   - (f) "Ken"

   Labial/Lingual
   - (g) "knee"
   - (h) "dough," "doe"

   Voiced/Voiceless
   - (i) "zoo"
   - (j) "cold"

Continued/Interrupted
    (k) "bee," "B," "Bea"   (l) "three"

Nasal/Non-Nasal
    (m) "me," "mi"   (n) "D"

Strident/Mellow
    (o)"sum," "some"   (p) "cheep," "cheap"

Appendix A
Differential Diagnostic Work-Up

Client: _____ Mother's occupation: _____
Age: __ years __ months (__/__/__) Father's occupation: _____
Complaint: " _____ ."

Etiological Factors

Environmental:

Second Language in Home [ ]¹ _____
Regional Dialect [ ]¹ _____
Idioglossia [ ]¹ _____
Poor Parental Model [ ]¹ _____

Sensory:

Audiometric Problems [ ]² _____
Visual Problems [ ]³ _____
Diadochokinetic Rates [p][ ]⁴ Greater than 3 per/second? _____
  [t][ ]⁴ Greater than 3 per/second? _____
  [k][ ]⁴ Greater than 3 per/second? _____
  [p–t–k][ ]⁴ Greater than 1 per/second? _____

Constitutional:

Socio–Emotional Maturity [ ]⁵%ile [ ] _____
Receptive Vocabulary [ ]⁶%ile [ ] _____
Structural Adequacy [ ]⁷ _____
  lips [ ]⁷ _____
  teeth [ ]⁷ _____
  tongue [ ]⁷ _____
  velum [ ]⁷ _____
  palate [ ]⁷ _____
  alveolar ridge [ ]⁷ _____
  thoracic cavity [ ]⁷ _____

Symptomatic Factors

Production:

Estimated Level–(Primitive-Vowel-Back/9-Semivowel-Continuant-
  Sibilant)⁸
Confirming Substitutions [ ]⁸ _____
Unexpected Substitutions [ ]⁸ _____

Retention: Auditory Memory [ ]⁹%ile _____

Discrimination: [ ]¹⁰%ile _____

Comments: (__/__/__)–date

References

Blache, S. An exploratory investigation of the use of multidimensional scaling in the perception of phonemic stimuli. Doctoral Dissertation, Ohio University, 1970. (*Dissertation Abstracts International*, 1971, *31*, 5014–B; *University Microfilms* No. 71–4783, 229.)

Blache, S. *The Acquisition of Distinctive Features*. Baltimore: University Park Press, 1978(a).

Blache, S. Recent findings concerning the use of minimal-pairs in articulatory diagnosis. *Occasional Papers on Linguistics*, 1978, *3*, 224–234, (b).

Blache, S. An examination of seven distinctive feature matrices using perceptual judgements. Paper presented at the Annual Meeting of the American Speech-Language-Hearing Association, Atlanta, Georgia, November, 1979.

Blache, S., DeMaio, L., and Brown-Harding, C. A minimal-pairs teaching technique in distinctive feature training. Paper presented at the Annual Meeting of the American Speech-Language-Hearing Association, San Francisco, California, November, 1978.

Blache, S., and Martin, C. The prediction of similarity judgements with a distinctive feature system and the relative frequency of occurrence of distinctive features in the English language. Paper presented at the Annual Meeting of the Speech Communication Association, Washington, D.C., December, 1977.

Blache, S., and O'Brien, M. A clinical prototype for auditory memory span. *Journal of Communication Disorders*, 1979, *11*, 519–527.

Blache, S., and Parsons, C. A linguistic approach to distinctive feature training. *Language Speech and Hearing Services in Schools*, 1980, *11*, 203–207.

Blache, S., Parsons, C., and DeMaio, L. The effects of three presentation rates on the measurement of auditory memory span as assessed by a modern clinical test. Paper presented at the Annual Meeting of the Speech Communication Association, Washington, D.C., December, 1977.

Blache, S., Parsons, C., and Humphreys, J. A minimal word-pair model for teaching the linguistic significance of distinctive feature properties. *Journal of Speech and Hearing Disorders*, 1981, *46*, 291–296.

Blache, S., and Rodd, J. Examining the reception/production controversy using a minimal-pairs task. *Illinois Speech and Hearing Journal*, 1979, *12*, 9–13.

Cairns, G., and Butterfield, E. Assessing language-related skills of prelinguistic children. *Allied Health and Behavioral Sciences*, 1978, *1*, 81–130.

Compton, A. Generative studies of children's phonological disorders. *Journal of Speech and Hearing Disorders*, 1970, *35*, 315–337.

Haas, W. Phonological analysis of a case of dyslalia. *Journal of Speech and Hearing Disorders*, 1963, *28*, 293–246.

Haas, W. Phonological analysis of a case of dyslalia. *Journal of Speech and Hearing Disorders*, 1963, *28*, 293–246.

Ingram, D. *Phonological Disability in Children*. New York: Elsevier, 1976.

Jakobson, R. Phoneme and phonology. In R. Jakobson (Ed. and Trans.), *Selected Writing Vol. I: Phonological Studies*. The Hague: Mouton, 1962 (originally published in Czechoslovakian, 1932).

Jakobson, R. *Child Language, Aphasia and Phonological Universals* (A. Keiler, trans.). The Hague: Mouton, 1968 (originally published, 1941, as *Kindersprache, Aphasie und allgemeine Lautgesetze*).

Kantner, C., and West, R. *Phonetics*. New York: Harper and Brothers, 1960.

Leopold, W. Patterning in children's language learning. In A. Bar-Adon and W. Leopold (Eds.), *Child Language: A Book of Readings*. Englewood Cliffs, N.J.: Prentice-Hall, 1971 (originally published 1953).

McDonald, E. *Articulation Testing and Treatment: A Sensory-Motor Approach*. Pittsburgh, Pa.: Stanwix House, 1964.

Miller, G., and Nicely, P. Analysis of perceptual confusions among some English consonants. *Journal of the Acoustical Society of America*, 1955, *27*, 338–353.

Oller, D. Infant vocalization and the development of speech. *Allied Health and Behavioral Sciences*, 1978, *1*, 523–549.

Olmsted, D. *Out of the Mouth of Babes*. The Hague: Mouton, 1971.

Poole, I. Genetic development of articulation of consonant sounds of speech. *Elementary English Review*, 1974, *11*, 159–161.

Singh, S. *Distinctive Features: Theory and Validation*. Baltimore: University Park Press, 1976.

Sommerstein, A. *Modern Phonology*. Baltimore: University Park Press, 1977.

Stark, R. Infant speech production and communication skills. *Allied Health and Behavioral Sciences*, 1978, *1*, 131–151.

Templin, M. *Certain Language Skills in Children*. Minneapolis: University of Minnesota Press, 1957.

Walsh, H. On certain practical inadequacies of distinctive feature systems. *Journal of Speech and Hearing Disorders*, 1974, *39*, 32–43.

Weiner, F. Systematic sound preference as a characteristic of phonological disability. *Journal of Speech and Hearing Disorders*, 1981, *46*, 281–285.

Wellman, B., Case, I., Mengert, I., and Bradbury, D. Speech sounds of young children. *Univ. Iowa Studies on Child Welfare*, 1931, *5*, 1–82.

Wickelgren, W. Distinctive features and errors in short-term memory. *Journal of the Acoustical Society of America*, 1966, *39*, 388–398.

Winitz, H. *Articulatory Acquisition and Behavior*. New York: Appleton-Century-Crofts, 1969.

5 Remediation of Speech Patterns Associated with Low Levels of Phonological Performance

Barbara Williams Hodson

During the past decade, the special needs and problems of children with the *most severe* speech disorders have begun to be recognized. Typically, these children have been enrolled in speech classes targeting "one-phoneme-at-a-time" for five to six years or more. The devastating effect of unintelligible speech patterns on educational progress cannot be ignored. The child who has a limited repertoire of speech sounds typically experiences great difficulty developing adequate reading, spelling, and phonics skills.

Although children with severe phonological disorders admittedly are low in incidence, they should not be underserved. Programs which were adequate for children with "mild articulation disorders" have not proved to be efficient for children with multiple substitutions and omissions. It is imperative that members of our Speech-Language-Hearing profession develop and continually refine accountable, individualized programs for all children with communication disorders, including the unintelligible child.

Contributions by applied phonologists such as Singh (1976) and Blache (1978) in the area of distinctive features, Compton (1970) in the area of phonological rules, and Ingram (1976), Hodson (1980), and Shriberg and Kwiatkowski (1980) in the area of phonological processes, provided new alternatives for analyzing and categorizing articulatory deviations. The identification of systematic patterns in child speech samples opened new vistas for planning more efficient remediation programs for children with highly unintelligible speech.

During the mid-1970s, an experimental phonological remediation program designed specifically for children with the most severe speech disorders was instituted at a midwestern university speech and hearing clinic. During the six years it was in existence, the program attracted over 100 children between the ages of three and eight years. They had been referred because they were considered to be "unintelligible" or "essentially unintelligible." Most of the older children had already received from one to five years of "phoneme-oriented" articulation training, and some of the younger children had been enrolled in language programs.

Evaluations of their phonological systems provided a framework for developing and implementing individualized remediation programs which resulted in rapid intelligibility gains. As new data were obtained from these children, new hypotheses were formulated and tested, and alterations were incorporated. The maximum time required to complete the remediation program (i.e., to become intelligible) for the most severe clients was 18 months. The remediation approach which is described in the ensuing pages represents the culmination of clinical research findings obtained from 125 highly unintelligible children. The approach, which is based on phonological principles, is facilitative and integrative in nature.

Salient Aspects of Clients' Case Histories

The only etiological characteristic prevalent in the case histories of these children was that many had experienced mild hearing losses at some time. Otological histories commonly included recurrent otitis media, as well as some instances of myringotomy surgery and PE tube insertions.

Four of the children had repaired cleft palates, three children had submucous clefts, one child had been diagnosed at the Mayo Clinic as having "severe developmental apraxia," and three children had educational placements in rooms for the mentally retarded. Although some children evidenced neurological "soft signs," such as poor coordination and balance, most of the children appeared to be "developing normally."

The children's socioeconomic backgrounds varied from professional to welfare families, and numbers varied from "only" children to eight children in one family. Eight pairs of siblings attended, including two sets of twins. Five of the children were black, and one was oriental. There were two-and-one half times as many males as females.

Expressive language samples were difficult if not impossible to analyze, but receptive language measures indicated that with a few exceptions, these children were functioning within normal limits receptively. The one commonality which all shared was that their speech had developed slowly. Typically, they produced few if any consonants prior to their third birthday. Patterns such as *Consonant-Vowel-Consonant* and *Consonant Clusters* were slow to emerge, as were certain classes of sounds, particularly stridents, liquids, and velars. At the time of onset of their respective remediation programs, the consonant repertoires for most of these children consisted of some of the following singletons /p b t d m n w/.

Assessment

Evaluation Procedure

The Assessment of Phonological Processes[1] (Hodson, 1980) was administered individually to each child. This instrument involves spontaneous naming of 55 common objects, body parts, or simple concepts. All American English phonemes are assessed at least twice—all prevocalically, and all postvocalically except /w, j, h/ in which instances only prevocalic productions can be elicited. Thirty-one common consonant clusters are also assessed in the 55 words. Administration time for each child required 15 to 20 minutes. (Although analysis of spontaneous connected utterances would have been desirable, this method was not possible due to the degree of unintelligibility of the speech samples. Most of the time the examiners were not able to identify the word being uttered without awareness of the stimulus object.)

All utterances were phonetically transcribed at the time of administration by the author and by one or more graduate students. In addition audio tape recordings were made which were utilized to verify transcriptions. Whenever discrepancies occurred among transcribers, the recordings were replayed until agreement was reached. Verified phonetic transcriptions were transferred from Recording Forms to the Analysis Forms (see Figures 1 and 2). The total number of instances of a child's use of each pattern was ascertained. Percentage-of-occurrence scores were derived for the major patterns by dividing the actual number of occurrences by the possible number of occurrences for each pattern. Means obtained from scores of the first 60 children currently serve as guidelines to assist the speech-language pathologist in identifying priorities for remediation (see Hodson, 1980).

Levels of Phonological Performance

Table 1 specifies four levels of phonological performance and gives examples of productions for each phonological pattern. In general, these levels coincide with intelligibility provided other factors, such as rate and voice, remain constant.

Level 0 (Unintelligible Except Via Gestures). The child with the most severe phonological disorder communicates to a limited extent via gestures and intonation pattern alterations during productions of vowels. Consonants are either nonexistent or limited to some sonorants.[2]

---

[1] The term "phonological process," is used here to simply describe a change which affects a whole class of sounds. For example, final consonants may be deleted (bed→/bɛ/) or clusters may be reduced (spoon→/pun/). The primary concern at this time has been to identify priority patterns that can be expeditiously remediated.

[2] Sonorant consonants include nasals, glides, and liquids /m, n, ŋ, w, j, l, r/.

BASIC PROCESSES

MISCELLANEOUS PROCESSES

Target	Production	1. SylRe	2. ClReOb	3. ClReSon	4. Pre→Ø	5. Post→Ø	6. Str→Ø	7. NonStr	8. Vel→Ø	9. VelFr	10. Pre→V	11. Post→D	12. GlRe	13. Back	14. Stop	15. Aff	16. Deaff	17. Pal	18. Depal	19. Coal	20. Epen	21. Meta
1. 'ɛkspleɪn																						
2. 'bæskɪt																						
3. bɛd																						
4. 'kændl																						
5. tʃɛr																						
6. 'kaʊbɔɪ,hæt																						
7. 'kreɪənz																						
8. θri																						
9. blæk																						
10. grin																						
11. 'jɛloʊ																						
12. dɑl																						
13. 'fɛðɚ																						
14. fɪʃ																						
15. 'flaʊwɚ																						
16. fɔrk																						
17. 'glæsɪz																						
18. glʌv																						
19. gʌn																						
20. 'hæŋɚ																						
21. hɔrs																						
22. 'aɪskjubz																						
23. 'dʒʌmproʊp																						
24. lif																						
25. mæsk																						
26. maʊθ																						
27. 'mjuzɪk,baks																						
28. noʊz																						
29. peɪdʒ																						
30. 'kwɔrtɚ																						
31. ruʒ																						
32. rʌg																						
33. 'sæntəkloz																						
34. 'skrudraɪvɚ																						
35. ʃu																						
36. slɛd																						
37. smuð																						
38. sneɪk																						
39. soup																						
40. spun																						
41. sprɪŋ																						
42. skwɝl																						
43. stɑr																						
44. strɪŋ																						
45. 'swɛtɚ																						
46. 'tɛləvɪʒən																						
47. ðæt																						
48. θʌm																						
49. 'tuθbrʌʃ																						
50. trʌk																						
51. tʌb																						
52. veɪs																						
53. wɑtʃ																						
54. 'joʊjoʊ																						
55. 'zɪpɚ																						
Totals																						

FIGURE 1. Analysis form. (Reproduced by permission of Interstate Printers & Publishers, Inc.)

| 22. /l/ → Ø | 23. → glide | 24. → vowel | 25. Other | 26. /r/ → Ø | 27. → glide | 28. → vowel | 29. Other | 30. Nasal → Ø | 31. Other | 32. Glide → Ø | 33. Other | 34. Vowel De | 35. Nas → A | 36. Vel → A | 37. Lab → A | 38. Alv → A | 39. /θð→ fvsz/ | 40. Fr Lisp | 41. t/tdnl/ | 42. → Lat | Other Patterns / Preferences |

SONORANT DEVIATIONS | ASSIMI-LATIONS | ARTICU-LATORY SHIFTS

THE ASSESSMENT OF PHONOLOGICAL PROCESSES
by
Barbara Williams Hodson

Name _____ Date _____ Examiner _____

PHONOLOGICAL ANALYSIS SUMMARY

Basic Phonological Processes

	Number of Occurrences	Possible Occurrences	Percentage of Occurrence
Syllable Reduction	_____	21	_____
Cluster Reduction			
Obstruent Omissions	_____		
Sonorant Omissions	_____		
Total	_____	35	_____
Singleton Obstruent Omissions			
Prevocalic	_____	38	_____
Postvocalic	_____	30	_____
Total	_____		
Stridency Deletion			
Omissions	_____		
Non-strident Substitutions	_____		
Total	_____	44	_____
Velar Deviations			
Omissions	_____		
Fronting	_____		
Total	_____	24	_____

Miscellaneous Phonological Processes

	Number of Occurrences
Prevocalic Voicing	_____
Postvocalic Devoicing	_____
Glottal Replacement	_____
Backing	_____
Stopping	_____
Affrication	_____
Deaffrication	_____
Palatalization	_____
Depalatalization	_____
Coalescence	_____
Epenthesis	_____
Metathesis	_____

(CONTINUED ON REVERSE SIDE)

FIGURE 2. Summary form. (Reproduced by permission of Interstate Printers & Publishers, Inc.)

Sonorant Deviations

	Number of Occurrences	Possible Occurrences	Percentage of Occurrence
Liquid /l/			
Omissions	_____		
Gliding	_____	10	
Vowelization	_____	3	
Other	_____		
Total	_____	13	_____
Liquid /r,ɝ/			
Omissions	_____		
Gliding	_____	12	
Vowelization	_____	14	
Other	_____		
Total	_____	26	_____
Nasals			
Omissions	_____		
Other	_____		
Total	_____	19	_____
Glides			
Omissions	_____		
Other	_____		
Total	_____	10	_____
Vowel Deviations	_____		

Assimilation Processes

	Number of Occurrences
Nasal	_____
Velar	_____
Labial	_____
Alveolar	_____

Articulatory Shifts

Substitutions of /f,v,s,z/ for /θ,ð/	_____
Frontal Lisp	_____
Dentalization of /t,d,n,l/	_____
Lateralization	_____

Other Patterns/Preferences

_____	_____
_____	_____

Circle each phoneme which was appropriately produced (whether or not it was the target).
/p b m w j t d n h f v s z ʃ ʒ ʧ ʤ k g ŋ θ ð l r ɝ/
Cross out each phoneme which could not be elicited with stimulation.

TABLE 1. Levels of Phonological Performance

LEVEL	PHONOLOGICAL PATTERNS	EXAMPLES		
0	No Obstruents	hat	→	/æ/, /wæ/
I	Syllable Reduction	basket	→	/bæ/
	Omission of Postvocalic or Prevocalic Consonants	hat	→	/hæ/, /æt/
		watch	→	/wɑ/, /ɑt/
	Cluster Deletion	spoon	→	/un/
	Fronting of Velars	gun	→	/dʌn/
	Backing	Santa	→	/hæŋ kə/
	Glottal Replacement	hat	→	/hæʔ/
	Prevocalic Voicing	cow	→	/gau/
	Prevocalic Devoicing	gun	→	/kʌn/
	Reduplication	basket	→	/bæ bæ/
	Vowel Deviations	bed	→	/bʌd/
	Idiosyncratic Rules	basket	→	/bæ wə/
II	Cluster Reduction	spoon	→	/pun/
	Stridency Deletion	soap	→	/oup/, /toup/
	Stopping	leaf	→	/dip/
	Liquid Gliding	red	→	/wɛd/
	Liquid Vowelization	chair	→	/tʃɛʊ/
III	/θð/ → /f,v,s,z/	thumb	→	/fʌm/, /sʌm/
	Frontal Lisp	soap	→	/s̪oup/
	Lateral Lisp	soap	→	/ɬoup/
	Tongue Protrusion /t,d,n,l/	doll	→	/d̪al/
	Palatalization	soap	→	/ʃoup/
	Depalatalization	shoe	→	/su/
	Affrication	shoe	→	/tʃu/
	Deaffrication	chew	→	/ʃu/
	Final Consonant Devoicing	page	→	/peɪtʃ/

The following may occur at all Levels except Level 0.

	Assimilation	spoon	→	/fpun/
	Coalescence	spoon	→	/fun/
	Metathesis	mask	→	/mæks/
	Epenthesis	black	→	/bəlæk/
	Diminutive	fork	→	/fɔ˞ki/

Level I (Essentially Unintelligible).

The child with Level I patterns frequently omits weak syllables. Some children reduce all multisyllabic words to monosyllables. Typically the children with Level I patterns have a limited repertoire of consonants. They may use consonants at the beginning *or* ending of words, but usually not consistently in both places. Thus CV or VC (Consonant-Vowel or Vowel-Consonant) productions occur, but CVC structures are limited or nonexistent. The most common omissions are final obstruents.[3] The majority of the children do produce final nasals. Sometimes these children omit specific classes of sounds prevocalically. For example, all voiceless consonants or all glides may be missing at the beginning of words. It has been observed that children who delete prevocalic consonants usually delete prevocalic clusters, and children who omit final consonants typically delete postvocalic clusters.

Another common Level I pattern is fronting of velars (substitution of an anterior consonant, most often /t, d, n/ for a velar /k, g, ŋ/). The contrasting Level I pattern, backing (substituting a velar or glottal phoneme for an anterior phoneme), is much less common, but seems to have a particularly devastating effect on intelligibility.

The remaining Level I phonological patterns have not been found to be as pervasive. Also, these patterns often reflect a child's individual preference. The first of these patterns, glottal replacement, involves substituting a glottal stop for the target phoneme. It is a particularly common phenomenon in the speech of children who are just becoming aware that there are final consonants. The second pattern, prevocalic voicing, involves substitution of a voiced cognate for the target phoneme. This pattern is much more common than prevocalic *de*voicing, which involves substitution of the voiceless cognate. The next pattern, reduplication, involves repeating a preferred phoneme or syllable. Vowel deviations have not been found to be as prevalent as consonant deviations. A few children did neutralize all vowels.

Some children demonstrated idiosyncratic or child-specific rules. A few had a particular phoneme preference. For example, one child substituted /h/ for all prevocalic consonants. Several children used a glide to initiate final syllables. One child substituted /l/ or /n/ for all prevocalic voiceless obstruents. While some children demonstrated a place preference for velar fronting or backing, usually producing the anterior phoneme in word-initial position and the back phoneme in word-final position, two children did just the opposite.

Level II (Sometimes Intelligible—depending on extent to which topic is known).

All of the 125 children who had been referred for *severe* speech problems evidenced *every* Level II pattern to some extent. However, 100% occurrence was not evidenced by every child. Also, as children progressed from Level I patterns, they evidenced Level II patterns. For example, many children functioning at Level I *deleted* clusters and *omitted* liquids, but as they improved, they demonstrated cluster *reduction* and liquid *gliding*.

Cluster reduction has been found to be a very common pattern even in the speech of the older child with a phonological disorder. It involves

---

[3] Obstruents are the voiceless consonants and their voiced cognates including stops, fricatives, and affricates /p, b, t, d, k, g, f, v, θ, ð, s, z, ʃ, ʒ, h, tʃ, dʒ /.

omitting one consonant in a two-consonant cluster and one or two consonants in a three-consonant cluster (whereas cluster *deletion* in Level I involved omitting the *entire* cluster).

Stridency deletion refers to omission of the strident target or substitution of a non-strident phoneme for one of the strident phoneme targets /s, z, ʃ, ʒ. t ʃdʒ, f, v/. Stridency deletion and cluster reduction have been found to be the major phonological patterns in need of remediation.

Stopping refers to the substitution of a stop consonant /p, b, t, d, k, g/ for any other consonant, most often for fricatives, but sometimes for nasals, glides, and liquids, as well. Although stopping frequently occurs concommitantly with stridency deletion, it has not been found to be as critical a target for remediation purposes. Also, it has been observed that even the most unintelligible children produced some continuant phonemes.

Other Level II patterns are liquid gliding, which involves substituting a glide (/w/ or /j/) for a prevocalic liquid, and liquid vowelization, which involves producing a true vowel for a postvocalic or syllabic liquid target. Liquid deviations are fairly common patterns and may still occur after all other Level II patterns have disappeared. However, approximately one-fourth of these children with severe speech disorders demonstrated good word-final /ɚ/ productions even at the very beginning of their remediation programs.

Level III (Generally Intelligible).   Sibilant alterations and substitutions of /f, v, s, z/ for /θ, ð / characterize speech samples of children functioning at Level III. Whereas the child functioning at Level I or Level II may have *omitted* sibilants and /θ, ð/ or have *substituted stops* for them, the child functioning at Level III approximated the target acoustically.

The most common Level III pattern is the frontal lisp which involves tongue protrusions during productions of some *or* all sibilants. In addition, the frontal lisp is often accompanied by tongue protrusions during productions of other alveolar targets. Such tongue protrusions generally have little or no effect on intelligibility and can rarely be detected on audio tape recordings.[4] The other major distortion of sibilant targets is the lateral lisp. Although it can be disconcerting, it does not particularly reduce intelligibility.

Several other Level III patterns also typically affect sibilants, although other classes are occasionally affected. Palatalization involves adding the palatal component while depalatalization refers to the loss of the palatal component. These patterns are fairly common as children sort out "shoe" versus "sue" distinctions. Affrication involves adding a stop element before a fricative, and deaffrication refers to deleting the stop. Children frequently use affrication and deaffrication when sorting out distinctions such as "shoe"

---

[4] Stridency is maintained in the frontal lisp, and it is often exaggerated by adults with frontal lisps. Thus the frontal lisp is not a /θ/ substitution for sibilants, since the /θ/ is quiet and non-strident. Very rarely does a child substitute /θ/ for /s/, and in such an instance, it would be a non-strident substitution rather than a frontal lisp.

versus "chew." Some children exhibit palatalization and affrication (and stridency addition) in place of a stop-plus-liquid consonant cluster target, such as /dʒin/ for "green."

The last Level III pattern, postvocalic devoicing, is very normal. It has been found that normally-developing children typically prolong the vowel, but most do not consistently voice word-final /z, ʒ, dʒ, b, d, g, v, ð/. For example, most intelligible preschool children typically say /peɪtʃ/ 'for "page" (Hodson and Paden, 1981).

Miscellaneous.   The following patterns may occur at all levels except Level 0. When a phoneme is produced more like another phoneme in the word than the original target phoneme, *assimilation* is said to have occurred. There are many different forms of assimilation, but the ones most often observed are labial, nasal, velar, and alveolar. *Coalescence* refers to producing a new phoneme in place of two target phonemes, and the new phoneme—although it is neither of the original targets—retains features of both. For example, in the production of /fun/ for "spoon," /f/ replaced the /sp/ and retained the stridency of the /s/ and the labialness of the /p/. *Metathesis* involves switching phonemes or syllables. *Epenthesis* occurs when a phoneme, which may be either a consonant or a vowel, is added. *Diminutive* refers to the addition of /i/ at the end of the words.

Intervention

Identifying Remediation Priorities

Every one of the children in this study needed to target stridency and consonant clusters at some time during their remediation programs, and the majority also needed to target liquids. Velars and final consonants were the next most common patterns needing remediation. Fewer children evidenced difficulty with these two patterns than with stridency, consonant clusters, and liquids. In addition, individual children needed to target various other patterns. For example, the "backer" needed to target alveolars rather than velars.

An initial clue for selecting target patterns for remediation involves identifying levels of performance. For example, a Level I pattern with a percentage-of-occurrence score greater than 40% may need to be targeted before a Level II pattern, even if the Level II pattern occurs 100% of the time. Level II patterns supercede Level III patterns, and the needs of the child functioning at Level 0 are the most basic.

There are many target options available for children functioning at Level 0 and Level I. For the child with no obstruents, stimulability probing is the most effective means of selecting optimal targets. For the child who produces some obstruents, probing is also important. In addition, comparison of the individual's phonological process percentage-of-occurrence scores with means obtained from a large group of children with phonological disorders[5] (Hodson, 1980) helps to "pull out" the pattern most "out of line," which is typically also the one most in need of being targeted first and the one which will provide the greatest likelihood for success.

Cycles for Facilitating Pattern Emergence

The common management practice of "staying" with each phoneme until a specified criterion level has been reached has not been found to be efficient for the child with numerous articulatory errors. A concept which has worked quite well for these children has been that of *cycles*. Individual phoneme(s) within a phonological pattern are targeted for approximately 60 minutes each during the first cycle. Many phonemes are "re-presented" during ensuing cycles. Groupings occur during later cycles, and the complexity level increases. For example, /sp/ might be presented during one session in Cycle I followed by /st/, /sm/, and /sn/, one per subsequent session. In Cycle II, /sp/ and /st/ might be grouped together, and /sm/ and /sn/ might be presented together the second period, and all four might be "re-presented" during the same session in Cycle III.

The length of each cycle depends upon the circumstances. At a university clinic, cycles typically last 12 weeks because of semester constraints, and summer cycles last six weeks. In the public schools, Cycle I is typically longest in order to individually present at least two targets for each deficient pattern before recycling. Reassessment between cycles is essential to ascertain which patterns are beginning to emerge and which need additional "doses." Typically, not much progress occurs during Cycle I. Rather, it lays the groundwork, and if the foundation has been properly laid, extensive progress occurs during Cycles II and III (Hodson, 1981).

Remediation Targets

Level 0. The primary remediation goal for the child functioning at Level 0 is production of consonants (any consonants) postvocalically and prevocalically. If the child omits sonorants as well as obstruents, nasals and glides may be the place to start. *Final voiceless* stops /p, t, k/, however, are usually fairly stimulable. Providing slight amplification via an auditory training unit

---

[5] When the goal is to identify priorities and to provide a direction for remediation programming, it is more useful to compare a client's scores with scores of others who manifest similar speech problems than to compare the scores with those obtained from a normative sample.

has been found to be a virtual necessity for stimulating consonant productions for the child functioning at Level 0, even when audiological evaluations have not identified any hearing loss. As soon as the children can produce three or four obstruents either pre- or postvocalically, they are ready for Level I programming.

Level I, Cycle I.　　For the child demonstrating significant syllable reduction processes, a "dose" of "syllableness" yields positive results. A week of targeting bisyllabic spondee words such as "baseball" and "football," followed by a week of three- and four-syllable utterances such as "baseball bat" and "football player," has been found to be highly effective as a "starter" to induce putting syllables and words together.

For the child who can produce VC or CV, but not CVC syllable shapes, the primary target would be CVC, or production of both a beginning and an ending consonant in a word. Words such as "pipe," "pup," "pop," and "peep," are usually fairly easy to elicit.

Children with the most severe speech disorders typically do produce nasals and glides. If, however, these are missing from the child's repertoire, then postvocalic nasals and prevocalic glides and nasals do need stimulation. Also children have been found to be more likely to produce prevocalic obstruents (although they may use substitutions) than postvocalic obstruents. If prevocalic obstruents are missing, they, of course, should be stimulated. Likewise, postvocalic obstruents, which are omitted most frequently, need to be targeted when deleted. Thus, for the child who is omitting singleton consonants, the classes of sounds affected must be identified. For example, if a child is omitting sonorants *only* prevocalically and obstruents *only* postvocalically, there would be no need to target prevocalic obstruents or postvocalic sonorants.

Final voiceless stops /p/ and /t/ (e.g., mop, boat) are usually easy to elicit (unless the child is a "backer," in which case final /k/ would be easier than final /t/). Two or three weeks of facilitation of final voiceless stops usually serves to "start" the emergence of final consonants.

For children who demonstrate that they can produce some CVC structures, but who substitute /t, d, n/ for /k, g, ŋ/, the next step would be facilitation of back consonants. Most children can produce /k/ in a word such as "rock" (although they typically will say /wɑk/ or /bɑk/). Prevocalic /g/ and /k/ would be the next target(s) (with no concern at this time about the presence of absence of voicing). There are very few appropriate initial /k/ or /g/ target words. The clinician must remember potential assimilation effects. Thus "cat," "goat," "candy," etc. would be inappropriate because of the regressive influence of the alveolar which may make productions of the initial velar terribly difficult during first cycle presentations.

Occasionally a child will be unable to produce a velar during the first cycle. In such instances, the clinician can stimulate for the final /k/, but production practice of the /k/ should, of course, wait until a later cycle when

/k/ is more facile. If the child has no back consonants at all, the /h/ or the /t / might be a useful vehicle to "break the anterior hold."

For the child who backs, the alveolars would need to be targeted. Usually the voiceless stop /t/ in the word-final position is easiest, followed by its voiced cognate /d/ in the initial position.

If a child demonstrates additional Level I patterns such as inappropriate voicing, glottal replacement, vowel deviations, or idiosyncratic rules, these need *not* be targeted during the *first* cycle, since it has generally been found that these patterns usually clear up spontaneously as children improve their listening skills and produce more appropriate consonants. However, if any are still existent by the third cycle, it would be appropriate to provide some minimal pair contrasting and awareness building (e.g., "pie" versus "bye" for prevocalic voicing or "bed" versus "bud" for vowel deviations).

The child who can produce two- and three-syllable words and *some* consonant-vowel-consonant combinations is ready to begin targeting Level II patterns. The "fronter" or "backer" will typically need another "dose" or two of velars or alveolars during ensuing cycles.

Level II, Cycle I.   The primary remediation targets of Level II are consonant clusters (CCV and/or VCC), stridency, and liquids. Most of these children substitute a stop for the continuant stridents as "tand" for "sand," and omit the /s/ in clusters as "tand" for "stand." It has been found to be more expedient to target /s/-clusters first for these children since their typical response when targeting a word such as "sand" has been "s:tand." Thus, rather than struggling to dispose of the intruding /t/ at the same time the child is learning to produce /s/ (and later having to "reteach" /s/-clusters), it is easier and more efficient to allow the stop to remain and to simply teach the child to make the /s/ prior to the stop. Later, when /s/ production is facile, it may be taught preceding a vowel.

For some children, initial /s/-clusters /sp, st, sm, sn/ are easiest, while for others final /s/-clusters /ps, ts/ are. For the "backers" /sk/ and /ks/ are, of course, easier than /st/ and /ts/. Plurals can be quite useful in teaching final /s/-clusters (e.g., "boats," "ropes"). Another useful syntactic tool is third-person singular verbs (e.g., "jumps," "walks"), which allow active participation while the child is learning to produce stridency at the end of words.

Before completing Cycle I, it is a good idea to provide a "dose" of prevocalic /l/ and prevocalic /r/ in order to lay the foundation for emergence of liquids. The target words need to be carefully chosen to avoid labial assimilation effects. Also, it is helpful during the introductory stage to pause between the liquid and the vowel and to prolong the vowel in order to dispose of the intruding /w/ (e.g., saying /ɚɑ:k/ is preferable to /ɚ:wɑk/). At this initial presentation the focus is elimination of the simplifying glide production rather than perfect production of a liquid.

The child's speech should always be reevaluated between cycles to ascertain which patterns are beginning to emerge and which need "re-targeting." The level of complexity increases during ensuing cycles. Also, groupings speed up the process and allow introduction of additional targets.

Level I, Cycle II (and Cycles III, IV, and V as needed). Usually final consonants do not need a second presentation, but velars typically require two or three presentations. By the third presentation, however, more difficult words can be incorporated, such as "cat" and "gate."

Level II, Cycles II and III, etc. The focus for Cycles II and III has generally been stridency and clusters (and to a lesser extent, the liquids). It may be appropriate by this time to present a week of prevocalic /s/. Other strident phonemes such as /f/ and /ʃ/ might also be introduced. One simple phrase that has been useful in facilitating generalization of stridency is "It's a _____." The first week it is presented with "non-/s/" words (for example, "It's a door."). The next week /s/ words are incorporated (e.g., "It's a spoon. It's a star"). Tactual cues and the auditory training unit serve to help the child sort out where the /s/ belongs.

During Cycle III more complex clusters are sometimes presented (especially for older children), such as liquid clusters, velar clusters, difficult /s/-clusters and three-consonant clusters (e.g., "tree," "glass," "mask," and "string"). It has been found that preschool children have demonstrated greater ability to generalize to the more complex clusters than have the older school-age children.

If additional recycling is necessary, the major targets are consonant clusters and liquids. It may also be appropriate at this time to target any residual Level I patterns (e.g., prevocalic devoicing) which may have persevered.

Level III. For the Level III child with a "mild" articulation disorder, the more traditional types of programming seem to be adequate. The primary remediation targets are /θ, ð/ and sibilants. However, a school-aged child will frequently be found who has not had sufficient auditory stimulation for liquids (particularly the /r/) during preschool years. Such a child will, of course, need to target the residual deficient liquid(s).

Remediation Procedures

The basic format for the remediation sessions was as follows:

Auditory Bombardment. Approximately two minutes of auditory stimulation (using an auditory training unit set at a low level) was provided at the beginning and end of each session while the child engaged in some quiet hand activity while listening attentively. The child did *not* repeat these words, and these words did not have to be carefully chosen.

Drawing Picture Cards. Following the auditory bombardment, the child drew (on 5×8-inch index cards) four or five pictures of *carefully chosen* words containing the week's target sound. The word was always written under the picture so that adults could identify the picture.

Experiential-Play Activities. The child participated in three or four simple activities each session, for example fishing, bowling, flashlight games. A picture card had to be named producing the target pattern correctly before taking a turn. Cues and assists were provided during the first productions, but were faded out as the child developed facility.

Probing. In order to determine the target for the next week, the clinician had the child repeat several words and then selected the easiest target within the deficient pattern. For example, if the pattern to be targeted was stridency in clusters, the probe words might have been "spoon," "star," "snake," "boats," and "ropes."

Auditory Bombardment. The session's target word list which had been read at the beginning of the session was again read to the child.

Home Program. This involved having the child name the picture cards once a day and also listening to the "auditory bombardment word list," which contained approximately 15 words using the target sound.

Variations. It has been found that children functioning below a three-year age level respond best when three-dimensional objects are used for production practice activities. Children functioning in the approximate range from three to seven years seem to enjoy drawing and naming pictures on their cards. Beginning readers can use a "mix" of printed words and pictures for words which they cannot read. Also, it has proven worthwhile to have the reader utilize the newly-learned phonemes in structured oral reading for five to ten minutes during each session. This seems to serve as an intermediary step to facilitate generalization for the older elementary child.

Fundamental Remediation Principles

Individualize Each Child's Remediation Program. A full phonological evaluation should precede development and implementation of the remediation program. Reassessment should occur at regular intervals to ascertain which patterns are beginning to emerge and which patterns need recycling. No two children out of the 125 who participated in this program followed exactly the same progression.

Facilitate Emergence of Patterns.   Targets should be presented in a systematic fashion based on phonological principles. Cycles provide a vehicle for presenting new targets, for grouping during later cycles, and for increasing the level of complexity as the child's performance improves.

Provide Auditory Stimulation.   A few minutes each day of auditory bombardment of the target phoneme(s) in words with the child *listening* and *not* repeating seems to help the child develop an auditory image for monitoring purposes. Children with phonological disorders can often recognize incorrect productions by other speakers, but they appear to lack adequate listening skills for monitoring their own speech productions. They seem to rely on kinesthetic images, which apparently match with their servosystem expectations. They need to learn new kinesthetic images during production practice at the same time that they are developing listening skills. Before generalization occurs, they need to be able to match auditory and kinesthetic images.

Incorporate Semantic Components.   It has been found that when children realize that there is a meaningful difference between the target and their production, the level of motivation tends to increase. For example, when children realize that the final strident phoneme makes a real difference between receiving "cookie" or "cookies," they typically will incorporate the /s/ more quickly than will those who simply "parrot" the strident phoneme multiple times.

Results and Summary

Phonological performance data were obtained from 125 children between the ages of three and nine years. All were considered to be highly unintelligible by parents and by professionals who referred them. Many of the children had already received speech-language services, but their parents and clinicians reported that progress was slow and that frustrations were occurring.

Table 2 provides data regarding client outcomes. Fourteen children were seen for purposes of evaluation and consultation only. They were unable to attend the university clinic on a regular basis. However, phonological information was provided to their local speech-language pathologists who had referred them.

Seventy children satisfactorily completed their phonology remediation programs and were dismissed because they were intelligible. The average time required was two semesters. The longest time needed by the most severe clients was 18 months.

Thirteen children had progressed substantially, but had not formally completed their programs by the July, 1981 program termination date. Seven children had been able to attend summer sessions only. Six children had

TABLE 2. Phonology Remediation Program Results
(June 1975 to July 1981)

CLIENT OUTCOMES	NUMBER OF CLIENTS
Program completions (3–18 months intervention)	70
Satisfactory progress	
Phonology program terminated before completion	13
Summer session attendance only	7
Program initiated, but not completed	
New 1981 clients	6
Families moved	7
Attendance/transportation problems	8
Evaluations/Consultations only	14
Total	125

barely begun their remediation programs by the July termination date. In addition, seven children were unable to complete their programs because their families had moved (four out-of-state, and three to distant points in the state). Eight children discontinued attending the university clinic due to various attendance/transportation problems.

The children who participated on a regular basis attended the university clinic once a week. The average length of their weekly lessons was 75 minutes. Many of the older children were also receiving programming in their local schools, typically, 20 minutes twice a week.

A number of the children were reevaluated periodically following dismissal from the university. In every instance, continuous gains in phonological development were noted. In fact, most of these children received no additional speech training.

The program which has been described in the preceding pages evolved over a six-year period. It was designed to serve the most unintelligible child clients and excluded children who were essentially intelligible.

Deficient phonological patterns were identified and systematically targeted with the emphasis being on *facilitating emergence* of speech patterns rather than on *perfecting* production of phonemes. The program was integrative as well as facilitative in nature, and the underlying goal was to expedite intelligibility gains.

References

Blache, S. *The Acquisition of Distinctive Features.* Baltimore: University Park Press, 1978.

Compton, A. J. Generative studies of children's phonological disorders. *Journal of Speech and Hearing Disorders,* 1970, *35,* 315–339.

Hodson, B. W. *The Assessment of Phonological Processes.* Danville: Interstate, 1980.

Hodson, B. W. Evaluation and remediation of phonological disorders. *Communicative Disorders: An Audio Journal for Continuing Education,* 1981, *6* (4).

Hodson, B. W. & Paden, E. P. Phonological processes which characterize unintelligible and intelligible speech in early childhood. *Journal of Speech and Hearing Disorders,* 1981, *46,* 369–373.

Ingram, D. *Phonological Disability in Children.* New York: Elsevier, 1976.

Singh, S. *Distinctive Features, Theory and Validation.* Baltimore: University Park Press, 1976.

Shriberg, L., & Kwiatkowski, J. *Natural Process Analysis.* New York: Wiley, 1980.

Index

The following pages present an index of major concepts (A) and procedures (B) referenced throughout this book. Readers will find guide reference to primary discussion areas relevant to each term. This is not a comprehensive list of terms nor are any authors indexed.

A: CONCEPTS

syllabic contexts,43
syllable, 9
  boundaries, 4, 9
  position, 9
  reduction, 18, 22
  reduplication of, 22
  structure, 18
syllableness, 109
syntagmatic, 77

target sounds, 6, 8, 10, 57
task, 25
therapeutic process, 78.
trade-off phenomenon, 24

uncoded processes, 45-46
underlying representation, 38, 43, 45, 56

variability, 14, 26
  in child speech, 15-23
  in procedures for
    data collection, 23-26
  in research findings, 14-15
velar preference, 17
vocables, 16
vowel deviations, 105
vowel lengthening, 19
vowel system, 84

word elicitation, 3, 71
word level approximation, 74
word position, 9

B: PROCEDURES

Assessment Data, 50
Assessment of Phonological Processes, 99
  analytic form, 99-101
  recording form, 99, 102-203
Auditory Bombardment, 111, 112

Carry-Over Training, 76
  connected speech, 76
  home situation, 76
Causal Correlates Data, 51-52
Cognitive-Linguistic Factors, 52
Consonant Inventory Sheets, 9
Criterion Levels, 73
Cycles for Facilitating Pattern Emergence,
  108-113
  length of, 108

Diagnostic Classification Form, 49
Differential Diagnostic Work-Up, 91, 94
Drawing Picture Cards, 112

Entry Points for Intervention, 55-56, 57
Experiential-Play Activity, 112

Grouping for Therapy, 68-70

Home Program 112
Homonymy Sheet, 9

Identifying Remediation Priorities, 107-108
Item and Replica Sheet, 9

Lexicon Sheet, 9

Mechanism Factors, 51-52
Minimal Pairs, 62, 64, 72, 77-78
  contrasting, 62-66, 90
  creating, 62, 70, 90

Natural Process Data, 50

Phonemic Contrasting, 27, 30
Phonemic Contrasting Board, 27, 28
Phonological Process Sheet, 9
Preparation Phase, 71
Presentation Phase, 71
Probing, 112
Psychosocial Factors, 52

Reassessment, 112

Segmental Data, 50
Smile, 75
Summary Sheet, 9, 49
Suprasegmental Data, 50

Teaching Distinctive Features, 71-78,
  90-91